www.harcourt-international.com

Bringing you products from all Harcourt Health Sciences companies ir ......ère Tindall, Churchi...... ...ngstone, Mosby and ......unders

○ **Browse** for latest information on new books, journals and electronic products

○ **Search** for information on over 20 000 published titles with full product information including tables of contents and sample chapters

○ **Keep up to date** with our extensive publishing programme in your field by registering with **eAlert** or requesting postal updates

○ **Secure online ordering** with prompt delivery, as well as full contact details to order by phone, fax or post

○ **News** of special features and promotions

If you are based in the following countries, please visit the country-specific site to receive full details of product availability and local ordering information

USA: www.harcourthealth.com

Canada: www.harcourt

Australia: www.harcou

D1344464

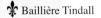 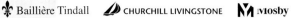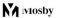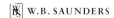

PICTURE TESTS
IN HISTOLOGY

Commissioning Editor: Timothy Horne
Project Development Manager: Jim Killgore
Project Manager: Frances Affleck
Designer: Erik Bigland

PICTURE TESTS IN HISTOLOGY

BARBARA YOUNG

BSc Med Sci Hons (St. Andrews), PhD Cambridge, MB BChir (Cambridge), MRCP (UK), FRCPA

Senior Staff Specialist in Anatomical Pathology, PaLMS Royal North Shore Hospital and Clinical Senior Lecturer in Pathology, University of Sydney, Sydney, Australia

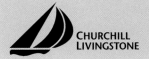

EDINBURGH LONDON NEW YORK PHILADELPHIA ST LOUIS SYDNEY TORONTO 2001
CHURCHILL LIVINGSTONE

An imprint of Harcourt Publishers Limited

⬗ is a registered trademark of Harcourt Publishers
Limited

First published 2001

ISBN 0443-06020-7

British Library Cataloguing in Publication Data
A catalogue record for this book is available from the British
Library

Library of Congress Cataloging in Publication Data
A catalog record for this book is available from the Library of
Congress

Note
Medical knowledge is constantly changing. As new
information becomes available, changes in treatment,
procedures, equipment and the use of drugs become
necessary. The author and the publishers have taken care
to ensure that the information given in this text is accurate
and up to date. However, readers are strongly advised to
confirm that the information, especially with regard to drug
usage, complies with the latest legislation and standards of
practice.

The
publisher's
policy is to use
**paper manufactured
from sustainable forests**

Printed in China

PREFACE

This book is written as a study aid for students of histology at all levels and is intended to be supplementary to standard texts and atlases. Each question includes a photomicrograph with an associated Type X (True/False) multiple choice question. The questions are designed to emphasise key points in histology, particularly functional aspects and general principles. The answers are accompanied by brief but comprehensive explanations, which should serve as a revision tool. The material examined is extensive, covering the full range of histology including ultrastructure of cells. The book is divided into 5 papers of 24 questions each and each paper contains both light microscopic and electron microscopic images.

In writing this book I have aimed to provide the student preparing for examinations with an alternative means of study to complement other methods. Repetitive study of lecture notes and texts is obviously important but it is easy to lose concentration and to assume that a vague familiarity with the material implies retention of key information. Approaching the material from the angle of practice examination questions may provide the necessary stimulus to get to grips with the nitty-gritty facts. It also provides practice at answering multiple choice questions, a widely used format for examinations. As a past examiner for both surgical Fellowship candidates and undergraduate medical students, I feel that the level of difficulty is suitable for both undergraduate and postgraduate students.

Barbara Young,
Sydney, Australia
September, 2000

ACKNOWLEDGEMENTS

I would like to thank Associate Professor John Heath of the Faculty of Medicine, University of Newcastle, NSW, for his great generosity in supplying all the electron micrographs for this book. The high standard of these images greatly enhances the overall quality of the book.

I would also like to thank all my colleagues of the Department of Anatomical Pathology, Pacific Laboratory Medicine Services (PaLMS) at Royal North Shore Hospital, Sydney. The staff specialists and registrars kindly donated material and the scientific and technical staff tirelessly cut and stained sections for photography. Without the patience and skill of the entire department, this book could not have been produced.

Alex Clarke is warmly thanked for her sterling efforts at the keyboard.

The photomicrographs were colour-separated and lettering added by the team at Chrome, North Sydney and I would like to thank the director Emmanuel Constantinou, Casto Pulgarin and all the others who made vital contributions to this work, often under very trying circumstances.

Lastly I would like to thank all my friends who provided support throughout the writing of this book and my two children Alex and Katie, who willingly tolerated cable TV and takeaway meals in the interests of histology students everywhere.

Barbara Young,
Sydney, Australia
September, 2000

CONTENTS

PAPER 1

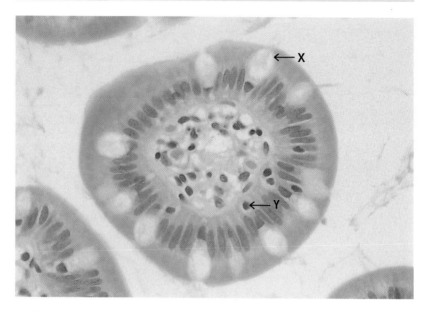

In this micrograph of a transverse section through a villus of the small bowel:

A   The main function of the epithelium is secretory.

B   The cells in the epithelium are held together by a junctional complex near the apex of the cell.

C   The cell marked **X** is a goblet cell.

D   The cell marked **Y** is most likely to be a lymphocyte.

E   The epithelium is a ciliated simple columnar epithelium.

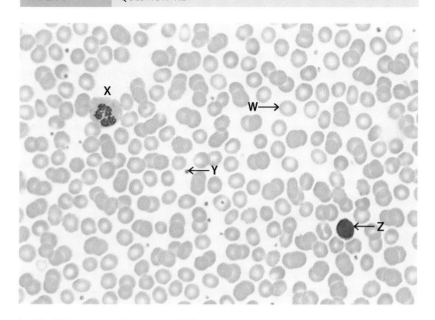

In this high-power micrograph of blood smear:

A   The cell marked **X** is a basophil.

B   The cell marked **Y** is derived from metamyelocytes in the bone marrow.

C   The cell marked **Z** is a circulating lymphocyte.

D   The cell marked **X** contains azurophilic granules in its cytoplasm.

E   The cell marked **W** is in the shape of a biconcave disc.

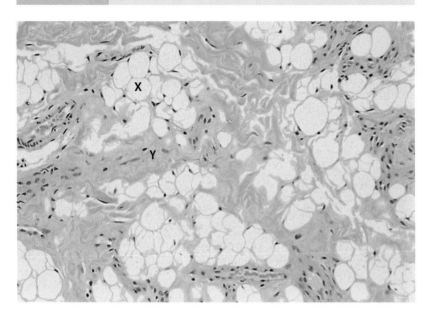

In this medium-power micrograph of supporting tissue:

A   The group of cells marked **X** have no nuclei.

B   Most of the cells in the area marked **Y** are fibroblasts.

C   The area marked **Y** consists mainly of collagen type I.

D   The area marked **X** characteristically contains few blood vessels.

E   The cells marked **X** are metabolically inert.

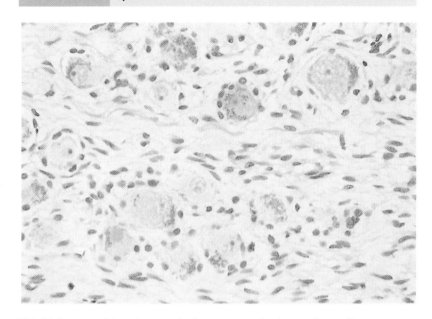

This high-power light micrograph shows sympathetic ganglion cells:

A   The pigment within the ganglion cell cytoplasm is melanin.

B   Melanin pigment is found in neurones of the substantia nigra.

C   Lipofuscin pigment is seen only in pathological conditions.

D   Most mammalian cells contain natural pigment.

E   Pigmented cells are normally found in the lung.

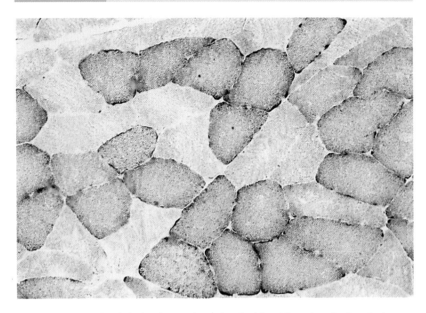

In this micrograph of skeletal muscle stained with a histochemical technique to demonstrate the mitochondrial enzyme, succinate dehydrogenase:

A   Densely stained fibres represent type II fibres.

B   Pale-stained fibres tend to derive energy from anaerobic metabolism.

C   Densely stained fibres are specialised for prolonged contraction.

D   Most muscles in humans consist of a mixture of fibre types.

E   The structure of the myofibrils in the type I and type II fibres is different.

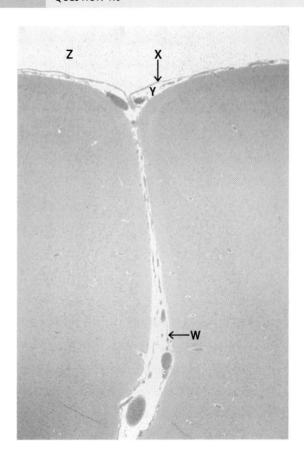

In this micrograph of the surface of the cerebral cortex:

A   The structure marked **X** is the pia mater.

B   The area marked **Y** contains medium-sized blood vessels.

C   Cerebrospinal fluid (CSF) circulates in the area marked **Y**.

D   The area marked **Z** is the extradural space.

E   The structure marked **W** consists of a single layer of ependymal cells.

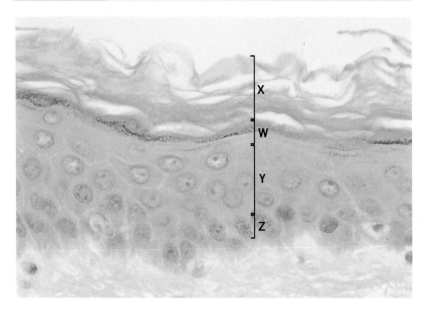

In this photomicrograph of skin:

A   The layer marked **X** consists of dead cells filled with keratin.

B   The cells in the layer marked **Y** have numerous desmosomes.

C   The cells in the layer marked **Z** divide to replenish the upper layers.

D   Most cells containing Birbeck granules are found in the layer marked **Z**.

E   The granules in the layer marked **W** are melanosomes.

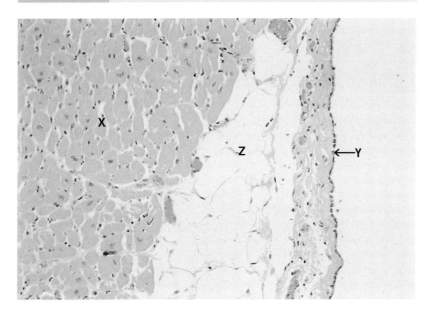

In this micrograph of the pericardium and underlying myocardium:

A   Purkinje fibres can be found in the area marked **X**.

B   The cells marked **Y** are endothelial cells.

C   The coronary arteries run in the area marked **Z**.

D   The cells in the area marked **Y** have long surface microvilli.

E   The cells in the area marked **Z** have abundant glycogen in their cytoplasm.

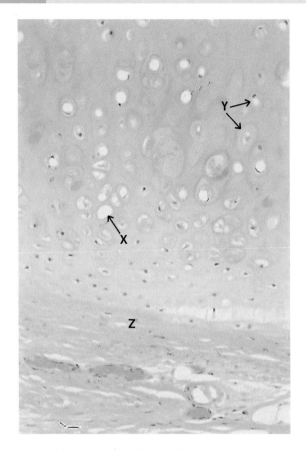

In this low-power micrograph of hyaline cartilage:

A   The space marked **X** is a small capillary.

B   The cells marked **Y** secrete the matrix.

C   **Z** marks the perichondrium.

D   The matrix is composed mainly of collagen type IV.

E   This type of cartilage is found in the larynx.

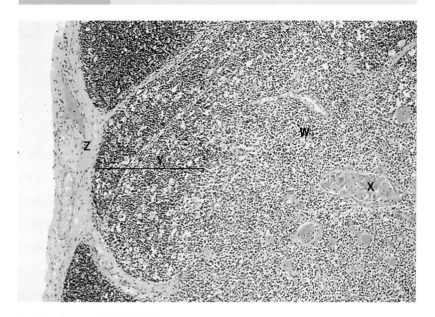

In this micrograph of fetal thymus:

A   The structure marked **X** is a Hassall's corpuscle.

B   The area marked **Y** is the main site of B lymphocyte maturation.

C   Thymic hormones are secreted in the structure marked **Z**.

D   In most individuals by the age of 25 the thymus has undergone total atrophy and is undetectable.

E   Antigen-presenting cells are found in the area indicated by **W**.

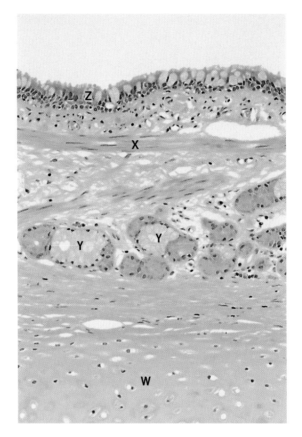

In this low-power photomicrograph of the wall of a primary bronchus:

A   The structure marked **X** consists of smooth muscle.

B   The structure marked **Y** is an apocrine gland.

C   The epithelium marked **Z** includes Kulchitsky cells.

D   The structure marked **W** is part of a C-shaped cartilage ring.

E   The structure marked **W** is composed of fibrocartilage.

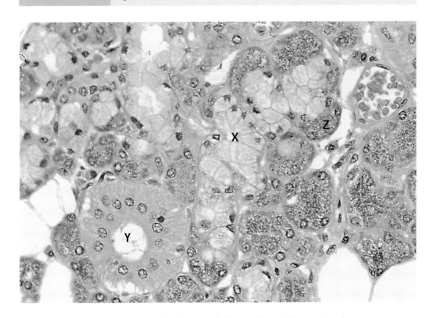

In this high-power micrograph of one of the major salivary glands:

A   The structure marked **X** is a mucinous acinus.

B   The structure marked **Y** is an intercalated duct.

C   The structure marked **Z** is a cluster of myoepithelial cells.

D   The gland is likely to be the submandibular gland.

E   The cells of the epithelium contain cytokeratin intermediate filaments.

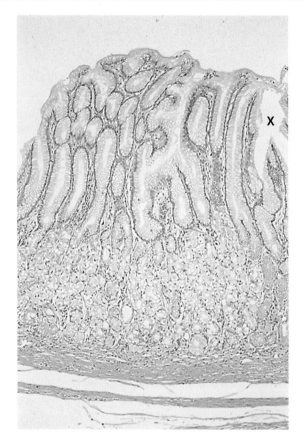

In this medium-power photomicrograph of the pylorus of the stomach:

A   The glands are lined by a mixture of mucous cells and peptic cells.

B   The structure marked **X** is a gastric pit.

C   Stem cells are found in the base of the crypts.

D   Gastrin is a major product of the mucous cells.

E   Gastric parietal cells may be present in small numbers.

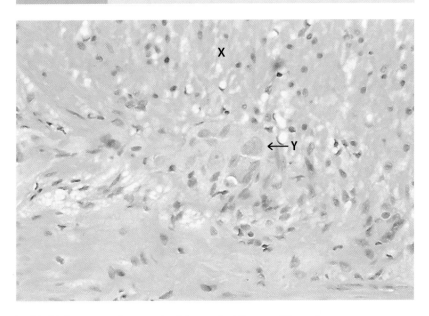

In this high-power micrograph of the wall of the small bowel:

A   The structure marked **X** is composed of skeletal muscle.

B   The structure marked **Y** is a cluster of sympathetic ganglion cells.

C   **Y** is part of Auerbach's plexus.

D   Activity of the parasympathetic nervous system enhances gut motility.

E   The cells of **Y** produce locally acting hormones.

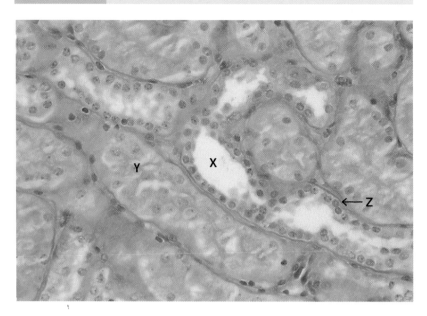

In this high-power micrograph of renal cortex:

A   The structure marked **X** is a distal convoluted tubule.

B   A major function of the structure marked **Y** is the secretion of antidiuretic hormone (ADH).

C   The cells lining the structure marked **X** are active in exchange of ions.

D   The structure marked **Z** is the tubular basement membrane.

E   The structure marked **X** is involved in the control of blood pressure.

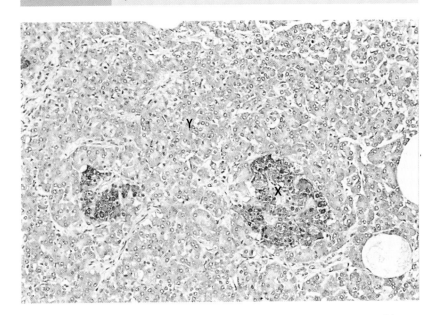

In this high-power micrograph of pancreas stained by the immunoperoxidase method:

A   The structure marked **X** is an islet of Langerhans.

B   The cells in the structure marked **X** contain dense core granules in their cytoplasm.

C   The cells that secrete insulin are arranged around the periphery of the cluster.

D   Secretion of hormones from **X** is via the intercalated duct.

E   The cells in the area marked **Y** produce glucagon.

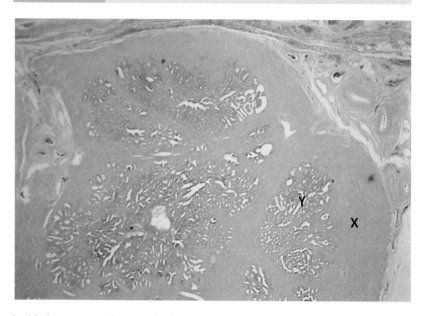

In this low-power micrograph of seminal vesicle:

A The lining epithelium is identical to prostatic epithelium.

B The structure marked **X** is a dense fibrous capsule.

C The epithelial cells secrete seminal fluid.

D The seminal vesicles drain into the ejaculatory ducts.

E The lumen marked **Y** is normally filled with spermatozoa.

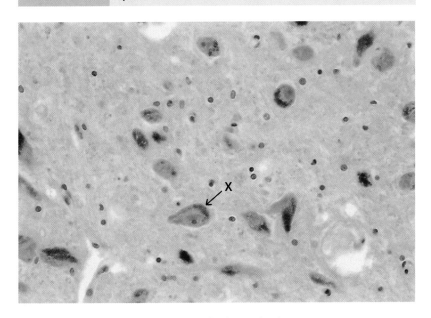

In this high-power photomicrograph of substantia nigra:

A   The cell marked **X** is a melanocyte.

B   The cytoplasmic pigment is melanin.

C   This section could have been taken from the brain of an infant.

D   A major neurotransmitter in the neurones of this area is dopamine.

E   This is a section of white matter.

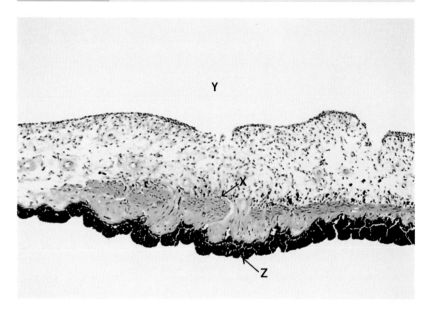

In this micrograph of the iris of the eye:

A   The structure marked **X** consists of smooth muscle.

B   The space marked **Y** is the posterior chamber.

C   The structure marked **Z** is a continuation of the pigmented epithelium of the ciliary body.

D   Melanocytes are plentiful in the stroma of the iris.

E   The iris is part of the uveal layer of the eye.

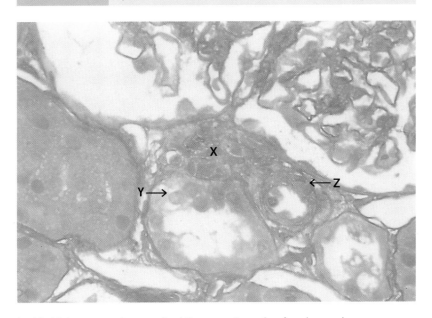

In this high-power micrograph of the vascular pole of a glomerulus:

A   Lacis cells are found in the area marked **X**.

B   The cells marked **Y** are the juxtaglomerular cells of the afferent arteriole.

C   Renin is produced by cells in the area marked **Z**.

D   Angiotensin II acts primarily on the cells in the area marked **Y**.

E   The cells marked **Y** are responsive to the sodium concentration in the urine.

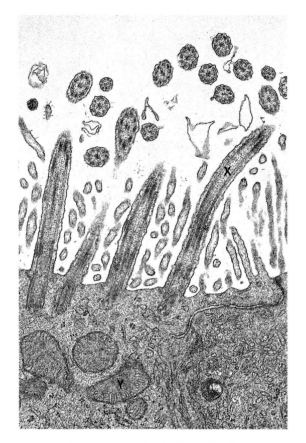

In this high-power electron micrograph of epithelial cells:

A   The structure marked **X** is a cilium.

B   The core of **X** contains doublets of myosin.

C   The core of **X** contains dynein arms.

D   The structure marked **Y** is an endocytotic vesicle.

E   The structure marked **X** has a central array of three microtubules.

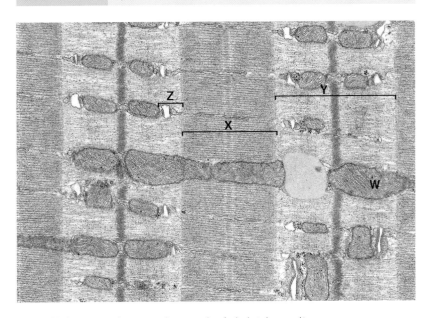

In this high-power electron micrograph of skeletal muscle:

A   **X** marks the I band.

B   The structure marked **Y** consists of actin and myosin filaments.

C   The structure marked **Z** is a tubular triad.

D   The structure marked **W** is a cell nucleus.

E   The width of the structure marked **Y** varies depending on the state of contraction of the muscle.

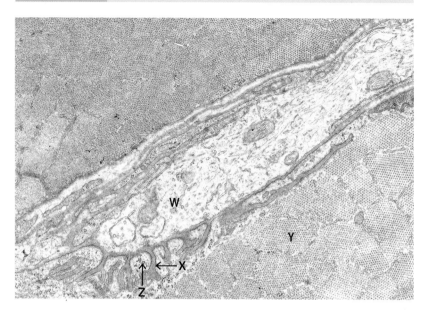

In this medium-power electron micrograph of a neuromuscular junction:

A   The structure marked **X** is a secondary synaptic cleft.

B   In the area marked **Y** myofibrils are seen in transverse section.

C   The structure marked **Z** is a group of synaptic vesicles.

D   The structure marked **W** is the nerve axon.

E   The enzyme acetylcholinesterase is found in the area marked **W**.

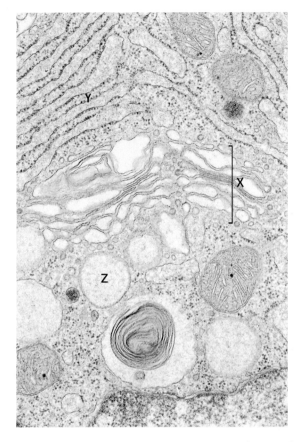

In this high-power electron micrograph of the cytoplasm of a protein-secreting cell:

A   The structure marked **X** is the Golgi apparatus.

B   The function of **X** is to modify protein structure.

C   The cisternae of **X** are surrounded by a double lipid bilayer membrane.

D   The structure marked **Y** is smooth endoplasmic reticulum.

E   The structure marked **Z** is a secretory vesicle.

A = False   The main function of this epithelium is absorptive. Although
            goblet cells are scattered throughout the epithelium to produce
            mucus, the majority of cells are **enterocytes**, which are
            absorptive cells responsible for uptake of nutrients from the gut
            lumen.

B = True   A **junctional complex** consisting of a **tight junction** (**zonula
            occludens**), an adhering junction (**zonula adherens**) and a row
            of **spot adhering junctions** (**desmosomes**) is found near the
            apex of each cell. The junctional complex links the cell to its
            neighbours and seals off the lumen of the gut from the
            intercellular space. These cell junctions are characteristic of (but
            not exclusive to) epithelial cells, allowing them to form a cohesive
            layer which acts as a permeability barrier.

C = True   The cell marked **X** is easily recognised as a goblet cell by the
            cytoplasmic clear area roughly in the shape of a drinking goblet.
            This clearing is seen in routine H & E stained sections. The
            cleared area is actually filled with **mucigen granules** containing
            mucus that is secreted onto the surface of the epithelium as a
            protective coating. The mucus consists of **mucopolysaccharides**
            and thus stains a strong carmine red colour using special stains
            for mucus such as the PAS stain. Goblet cells are found in other
            types of epithelium, notably respiratory epithelium.

D = True   Many normal epithelia contain a population of lymphocytes.
            These lymphocytes are typically found nestled between the bases
            of the epithelial cells as in this micrograph. In the gastrointestinal
            tract, most of these lymphocytes are T lymphocytes. They form
            part of the **gut-associated lymphoid tissue** (**GALT**), a subset of
            mucosa-associated lymphoid tissue (**MALT**) which defends the
            gastrointestinal tract against invasion by pathogenic organisms.
            These intraepithelial lymphocytes are found in greatly increased
            numbers in **coeliac disease**, a disorder of the small bowel that is
            probably of autoimmune aetiology.

E = False   This is a simple columnar epithelium with **microvilli**. Microvilli are
            found on many cells but the enterocytes of the small bowel have
            large numbers of microvilli (up to 3000 per cell). The microvilli
            cannot be seen individually with the light microscope but give rise
            to the **striated border** at the surface of the epithelium. The striated
            border is best seen here on the right side of the villus as a vague
            pink band. Microvilli may be slightly motile owing to their core of
            fine **actin microfilaments** but their primary function is absorptive.
            Microvilli greatly increase the area of the enterocyte membrane at
            the luminal surface thus greatly increasing the absorptive capacity.
            In contrast, cilia are easily seen at the magnifications achieved by
            light microscopy. Cilia are motile owing to the **microtubules** in their

core. They tend to beat in a coordinated fashion in the epithelium of the respiratory tract and the Fallopian tube where their function is to move mucus and ova respectively.

A = False   **X** is a **neutrophil** (neutrophil polymorph, polymorphonuclear neutrophil), so named originally because its cytoplasmic granules are neither basophilic (as in **basophils**) nor eosinophilic (as in **eosinophils**). The cytoplasm of neutrophils contains faint-staining granules. The nucleus is usually divided into multiple segments (hence 'polymorphonuclear') as seen in this micrograph. Eosinophils have bright orange-red cytoplasmic granules and a bilobed nucleus. Basophils are so packed with intensely basophilic (blue) granules that the nucleus is often obscured.

B = False   **Y** marks a **platelet**, which is derived from the **megakaryocytes** of the bone marrow. Platelets represent cytoplasmic fragments of the megakaryocyte and are anucleate. **Metamyelocytes** form part of the sequence of **granulocyte** maturation and come in three varieties: eosinophil, basophil and neutrophil metamyelocytes. All cells of the haemopoietic tissue of the marrow and of the blood are derived originally from a **pluripotent stem cell**. These cells divide to produce daughter cells, which give rise to all the different lineages of blood cells.

C = True   **Lymphocytes** are the second most numerous circulating white blood cell, neutrophils being the most numerous. Lymphocytes are easily recognised by their approximately round, intensely stained nucleus surrounded by a delicate rim of pale basophilic cytoplasm. Most lymphocytes in the blood are inactive and are en route to other sites. Hence the nuclear chromatin is densely packed (**heterochromatin**). Lymphocytes constantly recirculate between the blood, the lymph and the tissues. In the blood, a small proportion of larger lymphocytes are also found. These have a few cytoplasmic granules and are often called **large granular lymphocytes**. Some of these cells are activated B lymphocytes, while others are **NK** (**natural killer**) **cells**.

D = True   Neutrophils contain three different types of granule, which cannot be differentiated at this magnification. **Primary** or **azurophilic granules** are large lysosomes and contain the enzymatic machinery used for killing phagocytosed organisms. **Secondary granules** are smaller and can barely be resolved by light microscopy. Secondary granules store inflammatory mediators and are specific to neutrophils. **Tertiary granules** contain enzymes, such as collagenase, which help to break down damaged tissues during the process of tissue repair.

E = True   **W** marks an erythrocyte or red blood cell, the cell type responsible for the transport of oxygen to the tissues. In this particular staining method, the erythrocytes have a bluish coloration but more usually they stain a reddish-pink colour. Erythrocytes have a biconcave disc shape. This unusual cell shape provides a larger cell surface than a sphere of the same volume. Increased cell surface facilitates the diffusion of gases across the erythrocyte plasma membrane. It also allows greater deformability, which is useful when squeezing through narrow capillaries.

A = False   This tissue is **fibrofatty supporting tissue**, found in many sites of the body including the wall of the gastrointestinal tract and around many other organs. The cells marked **X** are **adipocytes** (fat cells) and, although the nuclei are difficult to detect, each cell has a flattened nucleus at one edge. The distorted shape of the nucleus is due to the presence of a single large lipid droplet occupying the bulk of the cytoplasm and compressing the nucleus and cytoplasmic organelles to the periphery of the cell. The only normally anucleate cells in the body are erythrocytes and platelets.

B = True   This is the collagenous component of supporting tissue and most of the scanty cells within it are **fibroblasts**, although there are also occasional lymphocytes, monocytes and mast cells. Fibroblasts are recognisable by their spindle-shaped nuclei and scanty cytoplasm, and produce the extracellular materials, including **collagen** and **glycosaminoglycans**, which constitute the bulk of this tissue.

C = True   **Collagen type I** is the main structural collagen found in fibrous supporting tissue of this type. This type of collagen is characterised by its tensile strength. Each collagen molecule consists of numerous **tropocollagen** molecules, polymerised by covalent bonds to form collagen fibrils. The fibrils are arranged into bundles that in turn are organised according to the stresses in the tissue. For instance in tendons the collagen bundles lie parallel to each other.

D = False   Adipose tissue characteristically is criss-crossed by an extensive capillary network. This capillary network is consistent with the high metabolic activity of adipose tissue (see E below).

E = False   Adipose tissue used to be thought to be metabolically inert, serving as an energy store and padding for the organs of the body. However, the lipid stored in adipocytes is constantly being turned over, with lipid being deposited or withdrawn from this 'energy bank' constantly, according to the nutritional state and rate of energy consumption of the individual.

A = False This pigment is **lipofuscin**, a pigment characteristically found in sympathetic, but not parasympathetic, ganglion cells. Lipofuscin accumulates in the cytoplasm of sympathetic ganglion cells with increasing age. Lipofuscin has a golden brown colour and is thought to be a degradation product of normal cell turnover, although this does not explain why it is found in some cells and not others.

B = True **Melanin** is the other major natural pigment and is found in the neurones of the substantia nigra, in the skin in varying amounts, and in the retina. In the skin and the retina the function of melanin is to absorb light, although this seems an unlikely explanation for its presence in the substantia nigra of the midbrain.

C = False Lipofuscin is found in many cell types in normal individuals. Apart from being in sympathetic ganglion cells, it is characteristically seen in liver and myocardial cells of normal individuals, usually as irregular brownish clumps close to the nucleus. Again in these cells its precise function is unknown. However, in pathological conditions where heart muscle undergoes atrophy, the amount of lipofuscin pigment increases, a condition known as **brown atrophy** of the heart.

D = False Most mammalian cells are not pigmented in thin histological sections and thus histological stains are required to see tissue under the microscope.

E = True It is rare to see lipofuscin in lung tissue and melanin is not a normal component of lung tissue. However, the alveolar macrophages of normal lung tissue usually contain pigment, which is mostly in the form of carbon particles. Carbon particles are present in the air we breathe, particularly those who live with atmospheric pollution, i.e. those of us who live in any town or city. The lungs of smokers contain even more pigment than those of non-smokers, for obvious reasons. As well as being found in the alveoli, these macrophages migrate to the hilar lymph nodes, which can easily be identified as such by the black, granular carbon pigment in the sinus macrophages. Pigmentation in alveolar macrophages is useful when assessing sputum cytology specimens. The presence of macrophages with cytoplasmic pigment in sputum smears confirms that the specimen is adequate, i.e. that it comes from the lungs rather than consisting of saliva.

A = False The densely stained fibres (**type I fibres**) are densely stained because they have more mitochondria and therefore more succinate dehydrogenase (a mitochondrial enzyme) than the paler fibres. These densely stained fibres are specialised for slower, continuous contractions and derive their energy for contraction from ATP produced aerobically by **Krebs' cycle**. Succinate dehydrogenase is one of the enzymes of Krebs' cycle.

B = True   The pale fibres are **type II fibres**, which are specialised for fast, short contractions. These fibres utilise ATP generated by anaerobic mechanisms and thus contain more cytoplasmic glycogen and fewer mitochondria than type I fibres. This difference can easily be seen in hens where the type II breast muscle is white because of the high glycogen content. Leg muscle is darker as it is mainly composed of type I aerobic muscle fibres.

C = True   As mentioned above, densely stained fibres contain more mitochondria with their content of succinate dehydrogenase. These fibres rely on aerobic metabolism for prolonged contraction.

D = True   Human skeletal muscles are composed of a mixture of fibre types because most muscles are required to perform rapid as well as continuous movements. For example, standing uses many of the same muscles as running. Standing requires prolonged continuous contraction and is thus fuelled by aerobic mechanisms. Running, in contrast, requires repeated short contractions but the muscles have a short recovery period after each step so that the lactic acid produced by anaerobic respiration can be cleared ready for the next contraction.

E = False   The myofibrils and their organisation in type I and II skeletal muscle fibres are identical. The mechanism of contraction is the same. The difference between the two types is in the source of energy used for contraction.

A = False   The structure marked **X** is the **arachnoid mater**. The **pia mater** is closely apposed to the surface of the brain and is difficult to identify in a low-power micrograph as here. Pia mater extends down into the **sulci** of the brain and surrounds the larger vessels entering the brain substance. Arachnoid mater bridges over the sulci. The arachnoid mater is a more substantial fibrous layer than the pia mater.

B = True   The arachnoid mater is separated from the pia mater by the **subarachnoid space**. This space contains the medium-sized vessels supplying the brain. The subarachnoid space is bridged by fine fibrous strands connecting the arachnoid and pia mater.

C = True   **Cerebrospinal fluid** (**CSF**) circulates continuously between the ventricular system and the subarachnoid space. CSF is produced by the **choroid plexus** found in each of the ventricles and circulates via three channels into the subarachnoid space. CSF is reabsorbed by **arachnoid villi** into the **superior sagittal venous sinus**. As there are no lymphatics in the CNS, extracellular fluid is thought to drain from brain tissue directly into the CSF, which thus acts as a 'lymphatic system' as well as a cushion against trauma.

D = False   This is the **subdural space**. The **dura mater** is not included in this micrograph as it usually remains adherent to the skull when the brain is removed. In life the arachnoid and dural layers are closely apposed to each other. However, trauma to the head may cause bleeding into the potential subdural space causing a **subdural haematoma** that may compress the underlying brain.

E = False   This is the pia mater, which is a thin layer of fibrous tissue. The facing surfaces of the arachnoid and pia mater are lined by flattened arachnoidal cells. In this micrograph there has been artefactual separation between the pia and the underlying brain thus making the pia more easily seen. **Ependyma**, a single layer of epithelial cells, is found lining the ventricles of the CNS.

PAPER 1	ANSWER 1.7

A = True   The superficial **keratin layer** or **stratum corneum** consists of dead cells, which are flattened, and have no nuclei or other organelles. These cells are filled with mature **keratin**. These cells have died by **apoptosis** (**programmed cell death**) and are constantly being replaced by maturing cells from the layers below. The keratin in the stratum corneum seems to be formed by some combination of the **keratohyalin granules** and **tonofibrils** found in the deeper layers. The keratin layer of the skin provides mechanical protection as well as being fairly impermeable to water.

B = True   The **stratum spinosum** or **prickle cell layer** is composed of cells which appear to be separated by a space bridged by thin strands of cytoplasm ('**prickles**'). The separation of the cells is probably an artefact caused by tissue processing. The prickles represent sites where adjacent cells are attached to each other by **desmosomes**. The large number of desmosomes in the cells of the skin gives the skin its resistance to abrasion.

C = True   Most cell division in the skin takes place in the **basal layer** or **stratum basale**. These cells represent fairly undifferentiated cells, which contain little **cytokeratin** in contrast to the more superficial differentiated cells. Cell division in this layer takes place at the same rate as loss of cells from the skin surface. Each cell takes about 25–50 days to mature from basal cell to desquamation at the skin surface.

D = False   The cells in the skin that contain **Birbeck granules** are **Langerhans cells**, which are present in all layers of the skin. Langerhans cells belong to the macrophage–monocyte lineage and function as **antigen-presenting cells** (**APC**). Langerhans cells are interspersed between the epithelial cells (**keratinocytes**) of the epidermis and have numerous processes, which extend between the keratinocytes. The Langerhans cell is a motile cell that is able to migrate to regional lymph nodes to present antigen acquired in the skin to lymphocytes. Langerhans cells are not easily identified in routine H & E sections.

E = False   The granules in the **stratum granulosum** or **granular layer** of the epidermis are **keratinohyalin granules**, which are an important component of the keratin of the stratum corneum. **Melanosomes** are found within **melanocytes**, the cells that synthesise the melanin pigment of the skin. Melanocytes are found scattered among the cells of the stratum basale.

A = False   **Purkinje fibres** are found in the subendocardial area of the myocardium of the ventricles. Purkinje fibres form part of the specialised conducting system of the heart, which allows coordinated contraction and relaxation during the cardiac cycle. Impulses arising at the **sinoatrial node** spread through the atria to the **atrioventricular node**. From here the impulse passes along the branches of the **bundle of His** to the terminal branches of the system, the Purkinje fibres. Rapid and coordinated nerve impulses lead to the entire ventricular muscle mass contracting simultaneously. Purkinje fibres have a similar appearance to cardiac muscle and probably represent modified myocardial cells.

B = False   **Endothelial cells** line the endocardial surface of the heart. These cells are **mesothelial cells**, which form the **visceral layer** of the **pericardium**. The **parietal layer** is formed by a similar layer of mesothelial cells. In normal individuals the two layers of the pericardium are closely apposed, separated only by a thin layer of serous fluid. This arrangement allows rhythmic movement of the heart within the chest cavity.

C = True   The coronary arteries and their branches run in the **subpericardial supporting tissue**, which cushions and supports the arteries.

D = True   The mesothelial cells of the pericardium, in common with mesothelial cells elsewhere, have long surface **microvilli**. These cells are simple cuboidal epithelial cells and rest on a basement membrane, which in turn is supported by a layer of fibroelastic supporting tissue.

E = False   These cells are mature **adipocytes** (**fat cells**), which form the bulk of the subpericardial supporting tissue. As in adipocytes elsewhere, the cytoplasm and nucleus are displaced by a large lipid droplet. Large amounts of glycogen in cytoplasm may also cause cytoplasmic clearing. However, glycogen does not give rise to the large well-delineated clear space characteristic of a lipid droplet.

A = False   Most hyaline cartilage is devoid of blood vessels. Exchange of oxygen and metabolites between blood and **chondrocytes** depends on diffusion through the matrix of the cartilage, which contains large amounts of water, the **water of solvation**. This empty space would normally contain a chondrocyte, which is not seen in this plane of section.

B = True   These cells are chondrocytes, which are found as single cells or small clusters embedded within the cartilage matrix. Chondrocytes produce the collagen and ground substance which make up the cartilagenous matrix and which are constantly being renewed.

C = True   The **perichondrium** is the thin layer of condensed fibrous tissue surrounding the cartilage. The spindle-shaped cells in this layer, which have the appearance of fibroblasts, are actually immature chondrocytes which can differentiate to form mature chondrocytes, e.g. during the growth of cartilage.

D = False   The matrix of hyaline cartilage is composed of ground substance and **collagen type II**. **Collagen type IV** is a major component of basement membranes. The ground substance of hyaline cartilage is composed of proteoglycan aggregates including **chondroitin sulphate**, **keratin sulphate** and **hyaluronic acid**.

E = True   Hyaline cartilage is found in the larynx, nose, costal cartilages, ears, trachea and bronchi, as well as many articular joints.

A = True   **Hassall's corpuscles** are clusters of keratinised epithelial cells, which, owing to the keratinisation of their cytoplasm, show marked eosinophilia (pink staining) with the H & E technique. Hassall's corpuscles are found in the **medulla** of the thymus and probably represent degenerate epithelial cells.

B = False   **Y** indicates the **cortex** of the thymus, which is packed with immature dividing T lymphocytes. The thymus is the organ where immature T lymphocytes, originating in the bone marrow, undergo division and maturation to produce clones of mature T lymphocytes. During this process the T lymphocytes acquire the surface markers which identify them as **T helper** or **T cytotoxic** *lymphocytes*. The T lymphocytes that pack the thymus are often called *thymocytes*. Occasional B lymphocytes, lymphoid follicles and plasma cells are found in the thymus but these are found in the perivascular spaces.

C = False **Z** marks the fibrous capsule of the thymus. This is a typical organ capsule composed of collagen with a few fibroblasts embedded in it. The origin of thymic hormones is unknown but it is most likely that they are produced by the *thymic epithelial cells*.

D = False Active thymus tissue is present in the mediastinum into old age. From the time of birth the thymus becomes progressively infiltrated by adipocytes, the process accelerating after puberty. However, microscopic examination of the fatty tissue of the anterior mediastinum in the elderly still reveals islands of easily recognisable thymus tissue. In a young adult, the organ is fairly easily recognised both macroscopically and microscopically.

E = True *Antigen-presenting cells* (*APC*) known as *thymic interdigitating cells* are found scattered throughout the medulla. Their function appears to be to present self-antigens (the individual's own body components) to the maturing T lymphocytes. Any T cells that are able to recognise these antigens become activated, thus identifying themselves as self-reactive T cells, which are then triggered to undergo apoptosis. Elimination of these cells, known as *clonal deletion* or *negative selection*, is a major mechanism whereby the immune system is prevented from reacting to the body's own components. Individuals in whom this mechanism fails, may develop autoimmune diseases such as *systemic lupus erythematosus* (*SLE*) or *autoimmune haemolytic anaemia*.

PAPER 1	ANSWER 1.11

A = True **X** marks the smooth muscle layer of the bronchial wall. Smooth muscle separates the *lamina propria* (above) from the *submucosa* (below). The smooth muscle in this micrograph appears to be branched because the muscle layer is discontinuous, with overlapping bundles of muscle fibres.

B = False The *submucosal glands* of the trachea and bronchi are *seromucinous glands*, similar in structure to the salivary glands. They secrete a mixture of mucous and serous secretions which moisten the airways and help to trap tiny particles in the inspired air. These secretions, along with the mucus secreted by the *goblet cells* of the epithelium, are swept upwards by the motion of the cilia on the epithelial surface and swallowed (mostly). This mechanism is known as the *mucociliary escalator*.

C = True   **Neuroendocrine cells**, known in the respiratory tree as **Kulchitsky cells**, are found in the epithelium of the respiratory tract. The Kulchitsky cells contain dense core granules in their cytoplasm and secrete a number of locally active hormones such as bombesin, serotonin and calcitonin, which regulate airway diameter among other functions.

D = False   In primary bronchi the cartilage takes the form of irregularly shaped plates, which become smaller in the smaller bronchi and disappear completely in the bronchioles. C-shaped cartilage rings are characteristic of the trachea, the open part of the C lying posteriorly and being bridged by the **trachealis muscle**.

E = False   The cartilage of the trachea and bronchi is **hyaline cartilage**, which is also found in the nasal septum, larynx, most articular joints and the costal cartilages. **Fibrocartilage**, which contains more collagen, is found in the intervertebral discs, the pubic symphysis, some articular joints and near joint capsules, ligaments and tendon insertions into bone.

A = True   The salivary glands are composed of a mixture of **serous** and **mucinous acini**. This is an acinus made up of mucinous cells, which, in this H & E stained preparation, have apparently clear apical cytoplasm owing to the mucigen granules that pack the apical cytoplasm. Serous cells have granular purple-stained apical cytoplasm (see below). Serous cells secrete a watery rather than mucinous fluid.

B = False   This structure is a **striated duct**. The very small **intercalated ducts** (not easily seen at this magnification) carry saliva from the acini to the striated ducts. The striated ducts modify the saliva by exchange of water and ions. Hence the striated appearance of the basal cytoplasm, which is due to numerous interdigitations of the basal plasma membranes of the adjacent cells, a feature which greatly enlarges the available membrane for ion exchange.

C = False   **Z** is a **serous demilune**, a feature seen in mixed salivary glands where both mucinous and serous cells are present. The serous cells, also seen in pure serous acini, are easily recognisable by their cytoplasmic content of enzyme-containing zymogen granules, which stain strongly by the H & E method. Pure serous acini are also seen in this micrograph. **Myoepithelial cells** are found flattened between the secretory cells and the basement membrane and are difficult to see in routine H & E sections. Occasional flattened nuclei of myoepithelial cells can be seen in this micrograph. Myoepithelial cells assist the expulsion of secretions into the ducts.

D = True   The **submandibular glands** consist of approximately equal amounts of serous and mucinous epithelium and produce saliva of intermediate consistency. The **parotid glands** are composed predominantly of serous acini and produce thin watery saliva, while the **sublingual glands**, consisting mainly of mucinous acini, produce a more viscid saliva.

E = True   The majority of the acinar cells in salivary glands (as in other glands) are epithelial cells characterised by cytokeratin intermediate filaments in their cytoplasm. The other cell type within the acinus is the myoepithelial cell, which typically contains both cytokeratin intermediate filaments and actin filaments. As indicated by the name myoepithelial, this cell type shows features of differentiation of two different lineages.

PAPER 1	ANSWER 1.13

A = False   The majority of epithelial cells lining the glands of the pyloric antrum are mucus-secreting cells. **Peptic** (or **chief** or **zymogenic) cells** are a feature of the bases of the glands in the body of the stomach and are absent in the pyloric antrum. Peptic cells in the body of the stomach secrete the enzyme pepsin, a proteolytic enzyme that begins the breakdown of ingested proteins into constituent amino acids.

B = True   The **gastric pits** of the pyloric antrum are longer than those in the gastric body, a feature that gives the surface of the mucosa a frond-like appearance. The mucus-secreting epithelial cells lining both the glands and the pits are similar to the neck mucous cells of the glands of the gastric body. The glands in the pyloric antrum are branched and coiled, in contrast to the straight simple tubular glands of the gastric body.

C = False   As in the body of the stomach, the **stem cells** are found in the neck of the glands. Stem cells, which are relatively undifferentiated cells, retain the capacity for cell division and divide at a constant rate to replace dead and dying cells throughout the gland. The daughter cells produced by the stem cell migrate up or down the gland and differentiate to form the various types of mature epithelial cells. Cell turnover proceeds at a constant rate in most epithelia but may be increased under different circumstances. For instance, during healing of a **gastric ulcer**, the epithelial cells must be produced at a higher rate to repair the defect in the epithelium. In most other tissues, with the possible exceptions of nerve and muscle tissue, undifferentiated stem cells are available for tissue growth, replacement and repair.

D = False   **Gastrin** is a product of the **gastrin** or **G cells** found scattered amongst the epithelial cells of the gastric antral mucosa. G cells are part of the *diffuse neuroendocrine system* and contain the characteristic *dense core granules* in their cytoplasm. G cells are not found in the body of the stomach but other neuroendocrine cells, with different secretory products, are found among the parietal and peptic cells in the body of the stomach. G cells cannot be identified at this magnification.

E = True   Although the acid-secreting parietal cells are most prominent in the body of the stomach, occasional parietal cells are also found in the pyloric antrum, especially near the junction with the gastric body.

A = False   **X** marks one of the smooth muscle layers of the bowel wall, part of the *muscularis propria*. Without knowing the orientation of the micrograph, it is not possible to determine which layer forms the *inner circular layer* and which is the *outer longitudinal layer*. However, no skeletal muscle is found anywhere in the muscularis propria of the gastrointestinal tract, except at the upper end of the oesophagus.

B = False   The structure marked **Y** is a cluster of *parasympathetic ganglion cells*. These are found at the interface between the inner circular and outer longitudinal layers of the muscularis propria as well as within the submucosa. Sympathetic nerve ganglia are not found within the wall of the bowel.

C = True   This ganglion and its associated nerve fibres along with many others similarly situated form *Auerbach's plexus*. The ganglia found in the submucosa make up *Meissner's plexus*. The postganglionic fibres of Meissner's plexus supply the muscularis mucosae, while the fibres of Auerbach's plexus supply the muscularis propria.

D = True   Parasympathetic activity enhances the motility of the gut, while sympathetic activity slows it. Sympathetic activity, as you will remember, is part of the *flight or fight response* that allows the body to take rapid action in appropriate situations. Thus sympathetic activity controls such factors as increased heart rate, dilatation of pupils and increased blood flow to muscles. Clearly in such a situation, evacuation of the bowels would be inappropriate, and sympathetic activity therefore decreases bowel motility.

E = False   The autonomic nervous system works in conjunction with locally produced hormones in the gastrointestinal tract. These hormones are produced by *neuroendocrine cells* that are found scattered throughout the mucosa. These two components, nervous activity and local hormones, act together with environmental factors such as the contents of the bowel to regulate the transit of food through the bowel.

A = True   In the cortex, **distal** and **proximal convoluted tubules** are intermixed. Distal convoluted tubules (DCTs) can be distinguished from proximal convoluted tubules (PCTs) by their smaller epithelial cells, lack of **brush border** (stained bright pink on the luminal margin of the PCT epithelium) and wider lumina. They also appear to be present in smaller numbers than PCTs because the DCT is shorter than the PCT. DCTs and PCTs are of course present in exactly equal numbers.

B = False   The **collecting tubules** and **ducts** secrete **antidiuretic hormone** (ADH), which regulates the water content of the urine. The PCT, which is marked by the letter **Y** in this micrograph, is the site of reabsorption of ions, glucose and amino acids from the plasma ultrafiltrate back into the bloodstream. This is facilitated by the profuse **microvilli** that expand the surface plasma membrane, and which are seen in this PAS-stained slide as a bright pink border along the luminal aspect of the cells, the brush border.

C = True   Active transport of ions is an important function of the DCT. In common with the PCT, the DCT has plentiful cytoplasmic mitochondria to supply energy for active transport as well as lateral plasma membrane interdigitations that expand the area of membrane available for active transport.

D = True   This staining method demonstrates basement membranes well and shows the **tubular basement membranes** which separate the tubules from the **interstitium**. The interstitium contains plentiful small capillaries into which the ions, glucose, amino acids and other substances pass to be returned to the general circulation.

E = True   The first part of the DCT forms the **macula densa**, which, together with the **afferent arteriole** and **extraglomerular mesangial cells**, makes up the **juxtaglomerular apparatus** (JGA). The role of the JGA is to detect changes in the blood pressure and sodium concentration in the blood of the afferent arteriole. The macula densa therefore acts as both a baroreceptor and a chemoreceptor. In response to lowered blood pressure and/or reduced sodium concentration, the JGA secretes **renin**, the first step in the **renin–angiotensin–aldosterone** mechanism for blood pressure regulation.

A = True   **Islets of Langerhans**, consisting of clusters of up to 3000 endocrine cells, are found scattered throughout the pancreas, and are most plentiful in the tail. Together the islets form an endocrine organ, the **endocrine pancreas**, which is responsible for maintenance of blood glucose levels. The major hormones secreted are *insulin* and *glucagon*.

B = True The cells of the endocrine pancreas belong to the general category of *neuroendocrine cells* and contain **dense core granules** in their cytoplasm. These granules or vesicles have an electron-dense core surrounded by a clear space, which is in turn surrounded by a membrane. The granules can only be visualised by electron microscopy but can sometimes be seen as a vague cytoplasmic granularity by light microscopy. Other neuroendocrine cells include the *C cells* of the thyroid, **adrenal medullary cells** and the cells of the **diffuse neuroendocrine system** such as the *G cells* of the stomach and the *Kulchitsky cells* of the bronchi.

C = False The cells producing insulin are found throughout the islet of Langerhans. They are known as **beta cells** and are generally demonstrated by immunohistochemical techniques using an antibody to insulin. **Alpha cells**, which secrete glucagon, are found around the periphery of the islet. Other cells in the islet (and scattered diffusely through the pancreas) secrete **somatostatin vasoactive intestinal polypeptide** (VIP) and **pancreatic polypeptide**.

D = False The islets of Langerhans constitute an endocrine organ and by definition secrete their hormone products directly into the blood. Each islet has a network of small capillaries lined by fenestrated endothelium into which insulin, glucagon and other hormones are released. The acinar tissue of the pancreas comprises the exocrine component of the gland and its secretions are discharged via *intercalated ducts* and the larger pancreatic ducts into the duodenum.

E = False These are acinar cells, which form the **exocrine pancreas**. Glucagon, like insulin, is a product of the islets of Langerhans. The acinar cells produce the digestive enzymes that are secreted via the duct system into the duodenum.

PAPER 1   ANSWER 1.17

A = False The lining epithelium of the **seminal vesicle** is different from prostatic epithelium. Seminal vesicle epithelium is a pseudostratified columnar epithelium with cytoplasm containing lipid droplets and lipofuscin. The nuclei are often quite variable in size and shape and these features are quite important in that seminal vesicle can sometimes be mistaken for **prostatic adenocarcinoma** in core biopsies of the prostate. The epithelium of the prostate, in contrast, consists of two cell layers: a tall

39

columnar luminal layer with pale cytoplasm and a flattened, sometimes incomplete, layer of basal epithelial cells.

B = False   The wall of the seminal vesicle consists of two layers of smooth muscle arranged (as in the gastrointestinal tract) into an inner circular and an outer longitudinal layer. This smooth muscle contracts during ejaculation, forcing seminal fluid into the ejaculatory ducts.

C = True   The seminal vesicle epithelium secretes approximately 85% of **seminal fluid**. This fluid carries the **spermatozoa** in the urethra during ejaculation and contains substances such as prostaglandins, vitamin C and fructose necessary for the function of the spermatozoa in the female genital tract.

D = True   Each of the paired seminal vesicles is a complex diverticulum of the **vas** (or **ductus**) **deferens**. The seminal vesicle and vas deferens joins to form the **ejaculatory duct**, which drains into the **prostatic urethra**.

E = False   Spermatozoa are stored in the **epididymis**, the coiled duct found on the posterior surface of the **testis**. The function of the seminal vesicles is secretory rather than storage. It is in the epididymis that spermatozoa undergo their final maturation and become motile.

PAPER 1	ANSWER 1.18

A = False   The cell marked **X** is a neurone, identifiable by its large nucleus, prominent nucleolus and plentiful cytoplasm. The cytoplasmic pigment is a unique feature of the neurones of the **substantia nigra** giving it a characteristic black appearance macroscopically. The neurones are embedded in a meshwork of axons and dendrites known as the **neuropil**. The small nuclei adjacent to the neurones are the nuclei of **glial cells** and demonstrate the very large size of the neurone cell bodies.

B = True   Melanin (**neuromelanin**) is the pigment found in the cytoplasm of the neurones of the substantia nigra. Its function is unknown but it may simply reflect a by-product of synthesis of **dopamine** from **DOPA** (dihydroxyphenylalanine). DOPA is also a precursor of melanin.

C = False   Melanin pigment is only found in substantial amounts in the substantia nigra of adults. In babies, the pigment is very scanty and it gradually increases with age.

D = True   Dopamine is the major **neurotransmitter** in this area of the brain. The substantia nigra is involved with the control of fine movement. In the condition known as **Parkinson's disease** there is a degeneration of the neurones of the substantia nigra and consequent reduction in the production of dopamine. This is accompanied by pallor of the substantia nigra when viewed macroscopically. In afflicted individuals there is a disorder of movement leading in some cases to almost total immobility. Fortunately, replacement therapy is available.

E = False   This is technically grey matter. The presence of many neurone cell bodies and consequently mainly unmyelinated axons (and dendrites) would give rise to a pale grey appearance in the absence of melanin, which actually makes the tissue appear black.

PAPER 1   ANSWER 1.19

A = True   The structure marked **X** is the constrictor muscle of the pupil (**constrictor pupillae**). This muscle, as its name suggests, constricts the pupil in response to nerve impulses from the parasympathetic nervous system. The constrictor pupillae muscle is arranged as a circumferential band of smooth muscle fibres, close to the free edge of the *iris*. The iris is dilated by the **dilator pupillae muscle**, which is much less easily seen. The dilator pupillae actually consists of **myoepithelial cells**, which form the basal layer of the two-layered epithelium on the posterior surface of the iris. The myoepithelial cells of the dilator pupillae are arranged radially and innervated by the sympathetic nervous system, thus causing the pupils to dilate.

B = False   The space marked **Y** is the **anterior chamber**. The eye as you will remember is divided into **anterior** and **posterior compartments**. The posterior compartment is divided from the anterior compartment by the **lens**. The anterior compartment is further subdivided into anterior and **posterior chambers**. The anterior chamber is anterior to the iris, while the narrower posterior chamber lies between the iris and the lens and its **suspensory ligament**. Both components of the anterior compartment are filled by **aqueous humor**, while the posterior compartment is filled by **vitreous humor** (**vitreous body**). The orientation of the iris is easy when you remember that the deeply pigmented epithelial layer is on the posterior surface.

C = True   The structure marked **Z** is the double layer of epithelium on the posterior surface of the iris. This is a continuation of the epithelial layer that lines the **ciliary body**. As mentioned above, the deep layer of this epithelium (the layer closest to the iris) consists of myoepithelial cells, which form the dilator pupillae muscle, while the superficial layer is highly pigmented. At this magnification the two layers cannot be differentiated from each other. In the ciliary body, it is the deep layer of the epithelium that is highly pigmented, while the superficial layer is non-pigmented.

41

D = True   Melanocytes are plentiful in the stroma of the iris. The deep
            pigmented epithelial layer contains approximately equal amounts of
            pigment in all individuals and the colour of the iris depends on the
            amount of melanin in the stroma. Blue eyed individuals have small
            amounts of melanin, whereas brown-eyed individuals have plentiful
            melanin.

E = True   The iris is one of three parts of the *uveal layer* of the eye. The
            eye consists of three layers. The outermost layer is the
            corneoscleral layer. The uveal layer is made up of the *choroid*,
            the ciliary body and the iris. The innermost layer is the *retinal
            layer*. The pigmented epithelium that covers the ciliary body and
            the posterior surface of the iris is a non-photosensitive
            continuation of the pigmented retinal layer. The photosensitive
            component of the retinal layer, the retina itself, ceases to be
            photosensitive at the *ora serrata*.

PAPER 1	ANSWER 1.20

A = True   This area is the *extraglomerular mesangium* and contains
            specialised mesangial cells known as *lacis cells* or
            Goormaghtigh cells. The exact function of these cells is not yet
            clear but it is thought that they participate in blood pressure
            control by modifying the diameter of the glomerular capillaries.
            This mechanism, known as the *tubuloglomerular feedback
            mechanism*, seems to involve the mesangial cells in the
            glomerular mesangium proper, which are able to contract and
            reduce the diameter of the glomerular capillaries, thus reducing
            glomerular blood flow.

B = False   This structure is the first part of the *distal convoluted tubule*
            (DCT) and the cells marked **Y** are a specialised segment of the
            epithelium known as the *macula densa*. Together the macula
            densa, the lacis cells and the *juxtaglomerular cells* of the
            afferent arteriole make up the *juxtaglomerular apparatus*, which
            is important in the control of blood pressure. The macula densa
            appears to be able to detect the concentration of sodium within
            the fluid in the lumen of the DCT. A reduction of sodium
            concentration increases renin production, which by means of the
            renin–angiotensin–aldosterone mechanism results in a
            compensatory increase in blood pressure.

C = True   The part of the wall of the afferent arteriole which is close to the
            macula densa of the DCT contains juxtaglomerular cells. These
            are modified smooth muscle cells that secrete renin, the first
            component of the renin–angiotensin–aldosterone mechanism.
            These cells are responsive to the chemoreceptor cells of the
            macula densa as well as acting as baroreceptor cells detecting
            blood pressure in the afferent arteriole.

D = False   The cells of the area marked **Y** are the epithelial cells of the macula densa (see above). These cells initiate the renin secretion which results in **angiotensinogen** being converted to angiotensin I and then angiotensin II. Angiotensin II raises the blood pressure by three principal mechanisms: constriction of peripheral blood vessels, promotion of aldosterone secretion from the adenal cortex and direct action on renal tubular cells promoting reabsorption of sodium and water from the DCT. The cells of the macula densa, although part of the DCT, have no active transport mechanism and are therefore not responsive to angiotensin II.

E = True   These are the cells of the macula densa and act as chemoreceptors for sodium in the urine (see above).

PAPER 1   ANSWER 1.21

A = True   **X** and all the similar structures at the cell surface in this micrograph are **cilia**. These are specialised structures found at the plasma membrane of epithelial cells in certain tissues (the bronchial tree, the epithelium of the nasopharynx, the Fallopian tube). Cilia are motile structures, which beat in a concerted fashion. In the bronchial tree, the beating of the cilia moves mucus up the bronchial tree. In the Fallopian tube, the beating of the cilia moves the ovum along the Fallopian tube towards the uterus.

B = False   The core of cilia contains nine peripheral doublets of **microtubules** as well as a central pair of microtubules (see E below). The peripheral doublets consist of a complete microtubule with a closely apposed incomplete tubule in the form of a C-shape. The microtubules arranged around the periphery are continuous with the microtubules of the **basal body**, which can be seen in some of the cilia in this micrograph. Near the top of the micrograph, some of the cilia are cut in transverse section and the nine doublets of microtubules are easily identified.

C = True   **Dynein arms** are found on each microtubule pair. Each of the complete microtubules has a pair of arms, extending towards the adjacent microtubule doublet. Dynein has **ATPase** activity and breaks down ATP to ADP, releasing energy in the process.

D = False   The structure marked **Y** is a mitochondrion. Several mitochondria are seen in this field, close to the surface of the cell. The mitochondria, as in other cells, produce energy in the form of ATP. This ATP is used as mentioned above as the energy source for movement of the cilia.

E = False   At the centre of each cilium, there is a central pair of complete microtubules. Together, the central pair of microtubules and the nine peripheral doublets are called the **axoneme**.

A = False   **X** marks the **A band**, which consists of **myosin** (**thick**) **filaments** and variable lengths of **actin** (**thin**) **filaments**. The A band has a central **M line**, which appears electron dense and is bounded on either side by a paler zone. The combination of M line and paler zone on either side is known as the **H band**.

B = False   The structure marked **Y** is the **I band** and contains only actin filaments with no myosin, myosin being restricted to the A band. The central dark line running along **Y** is known as the **Z line** where the actin filaments are attached. There is no overlap of actin and myosin filaments in the I band.

C = True   **Z** marks a **tubular triad**. These are found at the junction of I and A bands (depending on state of contraction of muscle). The tubular triad consists of a central flattened tubule of the **T system** with a pair of terminal cisternae of the **sarcoplasmic reticulum** arranged one on either side. The T system is a set of tubular extensions of the plasma membrane of the muscle cell, which ramifies throughout the cell. The lumen of the T system is therefore continuous with the extracellular space. The sarcoplasmic reticulum is a cytoplasmic system of membrane-bound tubules similar to endoplasmic reticulum in other cells. The sarcoplasmic reticulum contains concentrated calcium ions. When a depolarisation signal passes along the tubules of the sarcoplasmic reticulum, calcium ions are released from the sarcoplasmic reticulum into the surrounding cytoplasm (**sarcoplasm**) activating the contraction system of the muscle.

D = False   The structure marked **W** is one of many mitochondria seen in this electron micrograph. The mitochondria are arranged in a regular array in the I bands of the skeletal muscle close to the tubular triads. Mitochondria release the energy required for muscle contraction. The nuclei of skeletal muscle cells are arranged along the periphery of the cell and none are visible in this micrograph.

E = True   The I band becomes wider during muscle relaxation and narrower during contraction. During contraction, the actin and myosin filaments slide along each other (the **sliding filament theory** of muscle contraction). The length of the myosin filaments stays constant so that the A band stays constant in width, but as more of the actin filaments slide into the A band during contraction, the I band becomes narrower.

A = True   **X** marks a **secondary synaptic cleft**, one of many seen in this micrograph. The **synaptic cleft** is the space between the plasma membrane of the nerve ending and the plasma membrane or *sarcolemma* of the striated muscle cell. The secondary synaptic clefts are infoldings of the plasma membrane of the muscle cell. The receptors for the neurotransmitter, *acetylcholine*, are found at the margins of the secondary synaptic clefts. Acetylcholine is released into the synaptic cleft and binds to the receptors on the plasma membrane of the muscle cell thus activating contraction.

B = True   In the area marked **Y**, *myofibrils* can be seen in transverse section. You will note in this area that thick and thin filaments are visible in a regular array. This indicates that the section has gone through an *A band*. Note also the extensive network of membrane-bound tubules seen in the muscle cell. This represents the *T tubules* and *sarcoplasmic reticulum*. Occasional mitochondria are also seen between bundles of myofibrils as well as within the nerve fibre.

C = False   The structure marked **Z** is a group of free *ribosomes*. Close examination of the adjacent cytoplasm will show similar structures on the surface of membrane-bound vesicles, that is to say rough endoplasmic reticulum consisting of endoplasmic reticulum with ribosomes studded along its surface. *Synaptic vesicles* are not found in the cytoplasm of the muscle cell but are of course a feature of the *terminal bouton* of the nerve. Synaptic vesicles can be seen as hollow rounded structures on the nerve side of the synaptic cleft. The synaptic vesicles store acetylcholine ready to release it into the synaptic cleft when a nerve impulse reaches the terminal bouton of the nerve.

D = False   The structure marked **W** is the terminal bouton of the nerve, identifiable by its close association with the synaptic cleft and the secondary synaptic clefts. It is also identifiable by its high concentration of synaptic vesicles. The *nerve axon* is towards the right side of the micrograph and is continuous with the terminal bouton. Only a small portion of the nerve axon is included in this micrograph.

E = False   *Acetylcholinesterase* is found deep within the secondary synaptic clefts. Acetylcholinesterase breaks down acetylcholine so as to terminate the stimulatory signal received by the muscle.

PAPER 1	ANSWER 1.24

A = True   The *Golgi apparatus* consists of flattened *cisternae*, each surrounded by a lipid bilayer membrane. The cisternae are arranged in parallel with each other in a convex array, the concave face of which is usually orientated towards the nucleus.

Part of the nucleus can be seen at the lower right corner of this micrograph surrounded by a double lipid membrane. All cells contain one or more Golgi apparati. These are generally more numerous and more prominent in protein-secreting cells.

B = True   The main function of the Golgi apparatus is to modify and package proteins. The Golgi apparatus is usually in close apposition to the **rough endoplasmic reticulum** (**rER**, see D below). Proteins arrive in **transport vesicles** from the rER. The protein may either be contained within the lumen of the vesicle or embedded within its membrane. The transport vesicles fuse with the convex forming face (**cis Golgi network**). Protein modification takes place in a stepwise fashion with addition of carbohydrate side-chains. It is likely that only one specific type of carbohydrate residue is added in each cisterna of the Golgi apparatus, with the proteins being passed from one cisterna to another for sequential modification. On reaching the maturing face (**trans Golgi network**), the finished proteins are accurately sorted into secretory vesicles (see E below).

C = False   The cisternae of the Golgi apparatus are surrounded by a single lipid bilayer membrane similar to the plasma membrane, although containing different intrinsic proteins. The only structures within the cell that are surrounded by a double lipid membrane are the nucleus and mitochondria. In mitochondria there is an outer smooth lipid bilayer membrane, as well as the inner folded membrane, which makes up the **cristae** of the mitochondrion. Several mitochondria are identifiable in this micrograph.

D = False   **Y** marks rER that is found in almost all cells, but is particularly prominent in protein-secreting cells. rER can easily be identified by its outer coating of **ribosomes** attached to the surface. The ribosomes are attached to the cytoplasmic side rather than the luminal side of the rER membrane. rER is continuous with smooth ER and also with the outer membrane of the nucleus.

E = True   **Z** is a **secretory vesicle** leaving the Golgi apparatus. The secretory vesicle is likely to contain proteins for secretion as well as proteins embedded in its lipid membrane. Secretory vesicles migrate towards the plasma membrane. As they migrate, they become increasingly condensed and are then known as **secretory granules**. At the plasma membrane, the secretory granules fuse with the membrane, discharging their contents into the intercellular space. The fused membrane of the secretory granule with its intrinsic proteins becomes an integral part of the plasma membrane at the cell surface.

PAPER 2

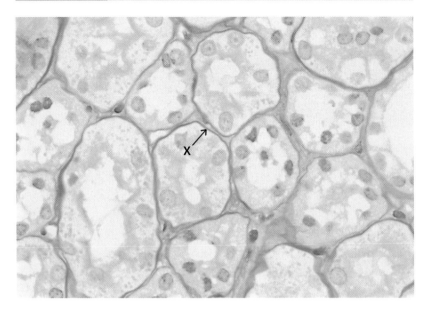

In this PAS-stained micrograph of human kidney the structure marked **X**:

A   Consists mainly of collagen type I.

B   Consists of three layers that may be seen by electron microscopy.

C   Allows passage of small blood vessels to supply the epithelium.

D   Is bound to the epithelial cells by hemidesmosomes.

E   Shows selective permeability.

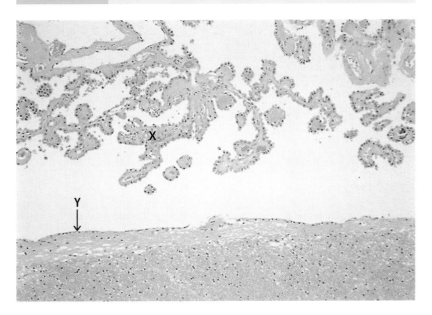

In this photomicrograph of the wall of one of the ventricles of the brain:

A   The structure marked **X** is found in the subarachnoid space.

B   The structure marked **X** produces cerebrospinal fluid (CSF).

C   The structure marked **Y** is composed of oligodendrocytes.

D   The cells of **Y** have surface cilia.

E   The cells of **Y** rest on a basement membrane.

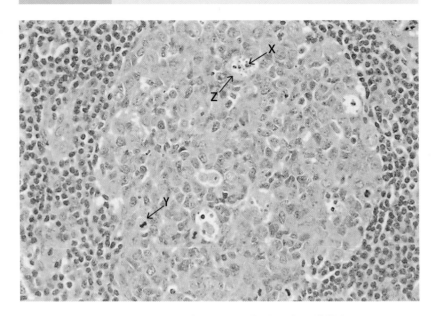

In this high-power micrograph of the centre of a lymphoid follicle:

A   The object marked **X** is a fragment of a cell nucleus.

B   The presence of the fragments marked **X** indicates that the tissue is necrotic.

C   The object marked **Y** is a cell undergoing meiotic division.

D   The appearance of the chromosomes in **Y** indicates that the cell is in the anaphase stage of division.

E   The cell marked **Z** is likely to have phagocytic properties.

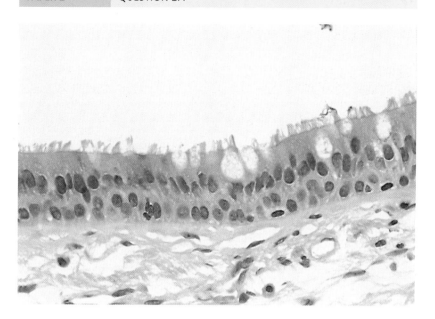

The epithelium shown in this high-power light micrograph:

A   Is likely to be found in the urinary tract.

B   Is of stratified squamous type.

C   Has microvilli on its surface.

D   Secretes mucus.

E   Consists of more than one cell type.

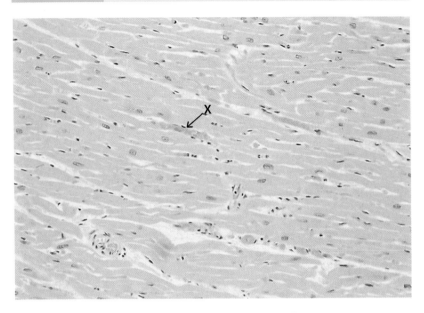

In this H & E stained photomicrograph of cardiac muscle:

A   The myocardial cells are joined at intercalated discs.

B   The individual cells are branched.

C   The myofibrils are arranged in a similar fashion to that in skeletal muscle.

D   The structure marked by **X** is a capillary.

E   The muscle cells form a syncytium.

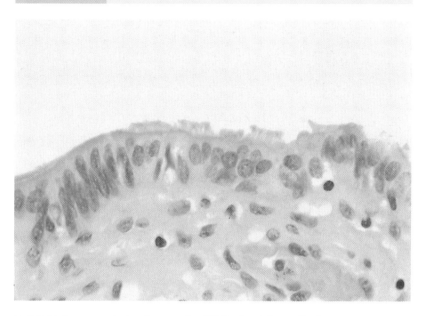

In this high-power photomicrograph of Fallopian tube epithelium:

A   The epithelium is of simple columnar type.

B   The surface projections are motile.

C   The surface projections contain a central core of actin intermediate filaments.

D   Each projection has a basal body at its base.

E   Dynein is a component of the core of the surface projections.

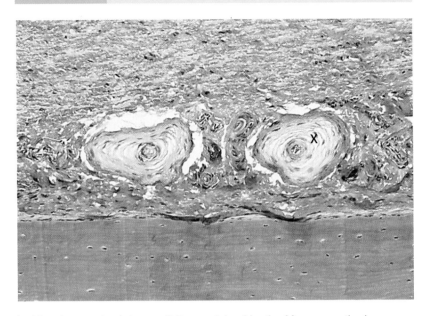

In this micrograph of deep soft tissue stained by the Masson method:

A   The structure marked **X** is a Meissner's corpuscle.

B   The central area of the structure marked **X** contains a myelinated nerve fibre.

C   The structure marked **X** is likely to be found in joint capsules.

D   The structure marked **X** is associated with Merkel cells in the epidermis.

E   The structure marked **X** is a sensory receptor for pressure.

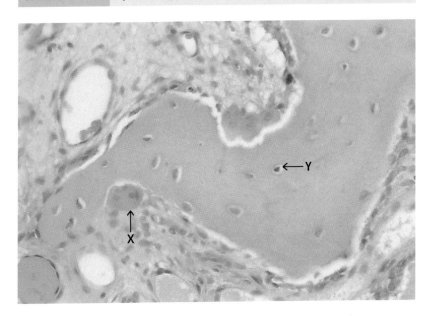

In this micrograph of bone:

A   The cell **X** is an osteoblast.

B   The cell marked **X** is prominent during bone healing.

C   The cell marked **Y** is an osteocyte.

D   The cell marked **Y** are stimulated by parathyroid hormone.

E   Bone becomes mineralised by deposition of hydroxyapatite crystals on unmineralised osteoid.

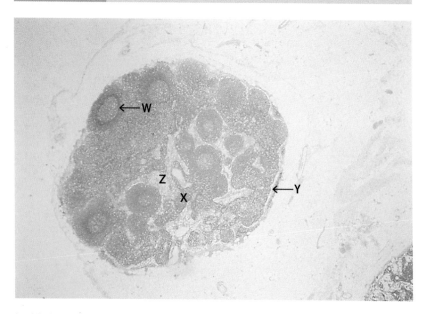

In this low-power micrograph of a lymph node:

A   The structure marked **X** is a medullary cord.

B   The structure marked **Y** is the subcapsular sinus.

C   The structure marked **Z** contains many T lymphocytes.

D   The structure marked **W** is a secondary follicle.

E   The structure marked **X** contains large numbers of plasma cells.

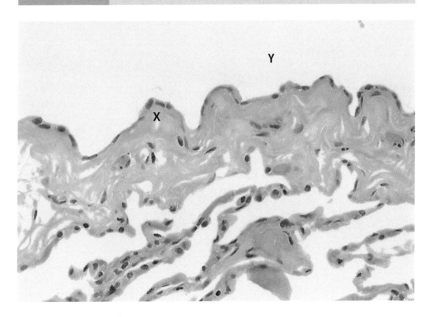

In this micrograph of lung:

A   The structure marked **X** represents the parietal pleura.

B   The space marked **Y** would be filled with air in life.

C   The surface cells of **X** have long surface microvilli.

D   The main lymph drainage of the lung is via the deep plexus of the pleura into the pleural space.

E   The supporting tissue of **X** contains plentiful elastin fibres.

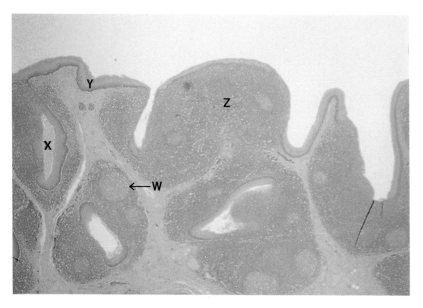

In this low-power photomicrograph of the posterior one-third of the tongue:

A   The structure marked **X** is a minor salivary gland.

B   The epithelium **Y** contains taste buds.

C   The tissue marked **Z** is part of Waldeyer's ring.

D   The structure marked **W** is a lymphoid follicle.

E   The structure marked **W** consists mainly of T lymphocytes.

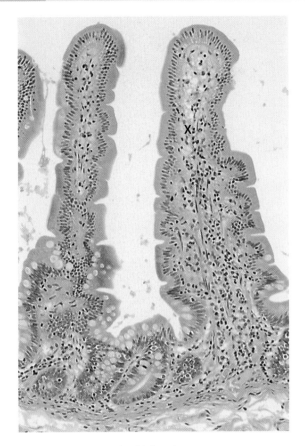

In this medium-power micrograph of jejunal mucosa:

A   The columnar cells lining the surface have large numbers of microvilli.

B   Submucosal glands secrete alkaline mucus throughout the length of the small intestine.

C   The cells at the bases of the crypts secrete antimicrobial substances.

D   The area marked **X** contains no lymph vessels.

E   Lymphocytes are found within the epithelium.

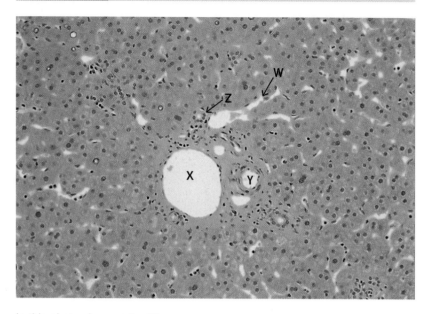

In this photomicrograph of liver:

A   The structure labelled **X** drains eventually into the hepatic portal vein.

B   The structure labelled **Y** drains eventually into the common bile duct.

C   The structure labelled **Z** is a bile ductule.

D   The structure marked **W** is a hepatic sinusoid.

E   The portal tract shown here is at the centre of the functional unit of liver structure known as the lobule.

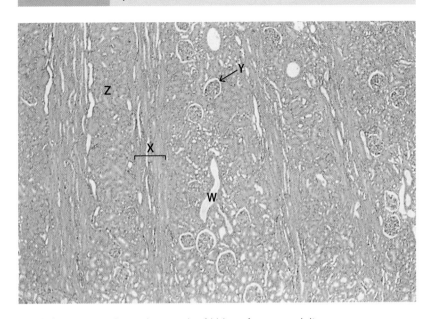

In this low-power photomicrograph of kidney from an adult:

A The cortex is divided into well-defined lobules.

B The structure marked **X** is a medullary ray.

C The structure marked **Y** is a renal corpuscle.

D The area marked **Z** is composed mainly of distal convoluted tubules.

E The structure marked **W** is an arcuate artery.

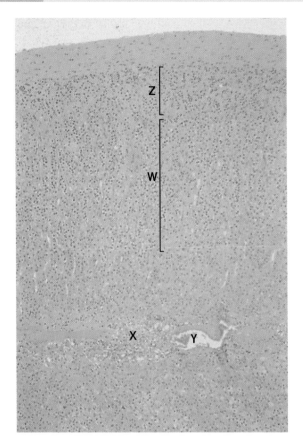

In this low-power photomicrograph of the adrenal gland:

A The zone marked **X** is responsible for the production of noradrenaline.

B The structure marked **Y** is the long cortical artery.

C The zone marked **Z** is the zona reticularis.

D The zone marked **Z** produces mainly aldosterone.

E The cells of the zone marked **W** contain plentiful smooth endoplasmic reticulum.

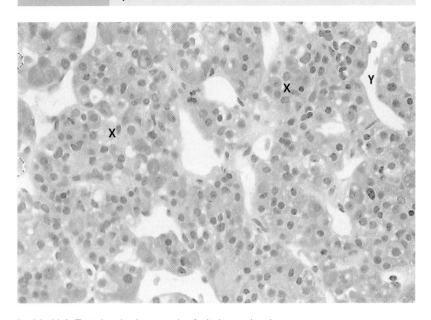

In this H & E stained micrograph of pituitary gland:

A   The cell clusters marked **X** consist of modified neurones.

B   The structure marked **Y** is a fenestrated capillary.

C   The cells in the areas marked **X** contain secretory granules.

D   All the cells in the areas marked **X** are responsive to luteinising hormone releasing hormone (LHRH).

E   Secretory products of the cells in the areas marked **X** include vasopressin (antidiuretic hormone).

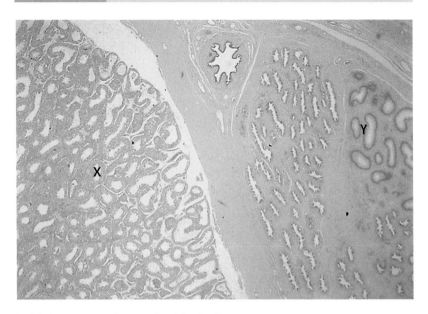

In this low-power micrograph of the testis:

A   The structure marked **X** is the rete testis.

B   The testis is surrounded by the tunica albuginea.

C   The structure marked **X** contains Sertoli cells.

D   Spermatozoa develop motility in the structure marked **X**.

E   The structure marked **Y** is the epididymis.

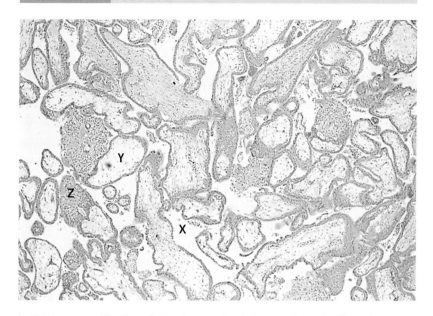

In this low-magnification photomicrograph of placenta from the first trimester of pregnancy:

A   The area marked **X** would be filled in vivo with fetal blood.

B   The structure marked **Y** is a chorionic villus.

C   The structure marked **Y** is lined on its outer surface by a double layer of intermediate trophoblast.

D   The structure marked **Z** is a bud of trophoblast branching to form a new chorionic villus.

E   The tissue in the central area of **Y** consists of mesenchyme.

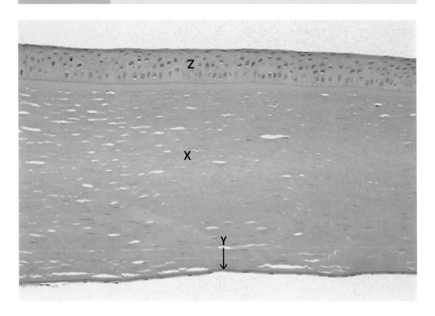

In this medium-power micrograph of cornea:

A   The area marked **X** is the substantia propria.

B   The structure marked **Y** is Bowman's membrane.

C   The structure marked **Y** has a lining of specialised endothelium.

D   The surface epithelium **Z** is of transitional type.

E   The cornea forms part of the scleral layer of the eye.

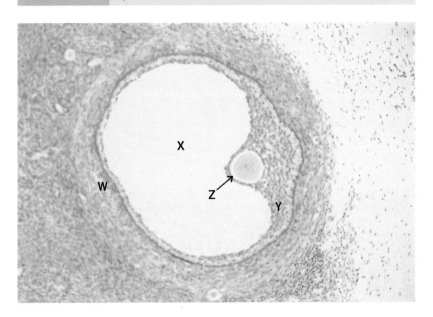

In this photomicrograph of the ovary:

A   The area marked **X** is the follicular antrum.

B   The cells in the area marked **Y** are theca cells.

C   The structure marked **Z** is the zona pellucida.

D   This is a Graafian follicle.

E   The area marked **W** is the zona granulosa.

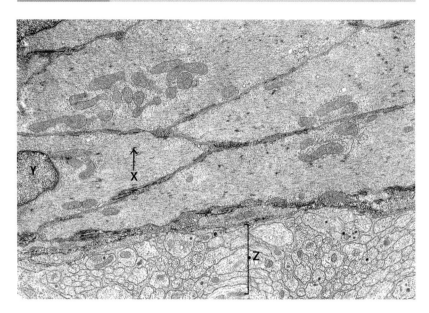

In this low-power electron micrograph of smooth muscle:

A   The structure labelled **X** is an anchoring density.

B   The structure labelled **Y** is a cell nucleus.

C   The cytoplasm is packed with filaments of actin and myosin.

D   The structure labelled **Z** is a small nerve bundle.

E   There are gap junctions between adjacent cells.

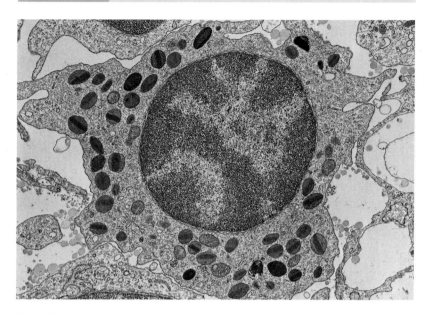

The cell in this high-power electron micrograph is derived from haemopoietic precursor cells and:

A   Is identifiable as a neutrophil.

B   Would normally have a bilobed nucleus.

C   Is responsible for secretion of immunoglobulins.

D   Has receptors for IgE on its surface.

E   Is important in the defence against parasites.

In the high-magnification electron micrograph of lung tissue on the facing page:

A   The area marked **X** represents the alveolar space.

B   The structure marked **Y** is the cytoplasm of an endothelial cell.

C   The cell marked **Z** is a mature erythrocyte.

D   The structure marked **W** is produced by type II pneumocytes.

E   The structure marked **Y** contains lamellar bodies.

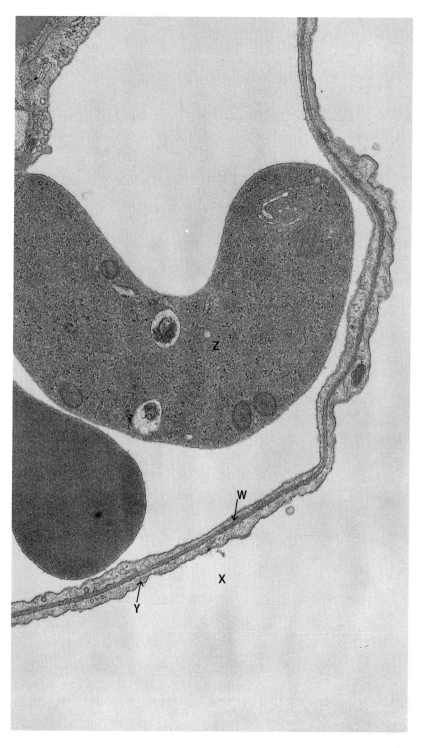

71

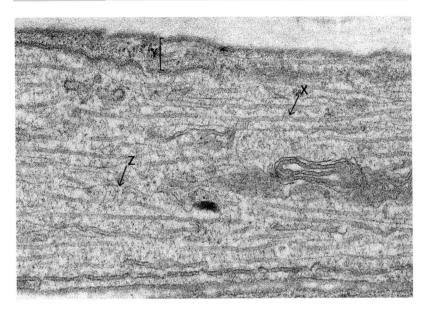

In this high-magnification electron micrograph of a nerve axon (longitudinal section):

A   The structure marked **X** is a microtubule.

B   The structure marked **Y** is the myelin sheath of the axon.

C   The length of **X** is variable.

D   The structure marked **Y** contains the same type of intermediate fibres as the axon.

E   The structure labelled **Z** is an intermediate filament.

A = False　This is the basement membrane of a renal tubule, the **tubular basement membrane**. Basement membranes contain mainly type IV collagen, which is unique to them. Type I collagen is found in other supporting tissues such as the dermis, tendons, ligaments, etc. The other components of basement membranes include **heparan sulphate**, **fibronectin**, **laminin** and **intactin**.

B = True　The layer of the basement membrane closest to the epithelial cells is a narrow electron-lucent layer, the **lamina lucida**. This rests on an electron-dense layer, the **lamina densa**, which is of varying thickness at different sites. The deepest layer, which becomes continuous with the surrounding supporting tissue, is the **lamina fibroreticularis**. Type III collagen predominates in the lamina reticularis.

C = False　All epithelia are devoid of blood vessels. Oxygen and nutrients diffuse into the epithelium from the capillaries in the adjacent supporting tissue, in this case the **interstitium** of the kidney.

D = True　**Hemidesmosomes** anchor the basal plasma membranes of the epithelial cells to the basement membrane and adjacent supporting tissues. On the cytoplasmic side of the plasma membrane, the hemidesmosome consists of a **plaque** of $\alpha_6\beta_4$ **integrin**. This plaque is linked to the **intermediate filaments** in the epithelial cell cytoplasm. The structure of the basement membrane adjacent to a hemidesmosome is different from that of the basement membrane elsewhere. At the hemidesmosome, the lamina densa is thickened and there is a thin electron-dense line in the lamina lucida due to the presence of anchoring filaments linking the integrins to the components of the extracellular matrix.

E = True　All basement membranes, including the tubular basement membrane shown here, exhibit selective permeability. In the case of endothelium, water and small molecules pass freely into surrounding tissues but larger molecules such as larger plasma proteins are contained within the vessel lumen. In the renal glomerulus, the selective permeability of the **glomerular basement membrane** is crucial to the formation of an ultrafiltrate of plasma. This function is enhanced by the highly specialised **podocytes** (epithelial cells) which contribute to the permeability barrier.

A = False　The structure marked **X** is the **choroid plexus**, which is found within all four of the **ventricles** of the central nervous system. The choroid plexus consists of a tangle of wide-calibre capillaries surrounded on their outer surface by a layer of modified *ependymal cells*. In life, the choroid plexus would be surrounded by *cerebrospinal fluid* (*CSF*).

B = True   The function of the choroid plexus is to produce CSF. CSF is produced constantly into the ventricles of the central nervous system and circulates through the *subarachnoid space* where it is reabsorbed into the *superior sagittal venous sinus*. Secretion of CSF occurs by active transport of sodium ions by the ependymal cells lining the choroid plexus into the surrounding space. The sodium ions are followed by water, which moves passively from the capillaries into the CSF. In accordance with this active transport function, the ependymal cells lining the choroid plexus have plentiful long microvilli and contain large numbers of mitochondria to provide energy for active transport.

C = False   **Y** marks the *ependyma* lining the ventricle. Ependymal cells are a form of modified epithelium which have a low columnar or cuboidal shape. Ependyma lines the ventricles and spinal canal. The ependymal cells are tightly bound at their luminal surface by *junctional complexes*. As you will remember, junctional complexes are made up of three structures, occluding junctions (*zonula occludens*), adhering junctions (*zonula adherens*) and *desmosomes*.

D = True   Ependymal cells have both cilia and microvilli. Cilia as in other epithelial structures contain microtubule doublets running along the length of the cilium. Cilia are motile structures and may have a function in moving CSF through the ventricles of the CNS. Microvilli are not generally motile and may have absorptive and secretory functions.

E = False   In contrast with almost all other epithelia, the ependyma lining the ventricles and spinal canal has no basement membrane. Instead the bases of the cells form fine branches, which interdigitate with the processes of the *astrocytes* in the underlying brain tissue.

PAPER 2   ANSWER 2.3

A = True   These darkly stained fragments are known as *apoptotic bodies*. They represent the remains of the nucleus of a cell that has undergone *apoptosis*. In the germinal centre of a lymphoid follicle as shown here, many cells undergo apoptosis. During the response to antigen, rapidly dividing lymphocytes undergo many random alterations to the DNA of their immunoglobulin genes (*mutations*). Some of the resulting cells are able to produce functioning antibodies and are allowed to continue division and maturation to produce clones of plasma cells. Other cells resulting from these mutational events are defective in some way and are induced to die by apoptosis. The advantage of the frequent mutations at this stage is that a great variety of immunoglobulin specificities is produced, some of which may be highly effective at dealing with the invading organism.

B = False **Necrosis**, which is almost always pathological, is characterised by death of whole areas of tissue. Necrotic tissue, such as is seen in the myocardium after **myocardial infarction**, usually excites an **inflammatory response**. Apoptosis, as seen in this micrograph, is characterised by the death of individual cells. The signals leading to apoptosis are varied, but the 'final common pathway' involves fragmentation of the chromosomes and eventual disintegration of the nucleus. The adjacent cells are usually entirely normal and there is no inflammatory response to this process. Apoptosis occurs in normal tissues (e.g. lymphocytes responding to antigen, during fetal development, during normal menstrual cycles) as well as in certain pathological situations.

C = False Only germ cells in the gonads divide by meiosis. Therefore, by definition, this cell is dividing by mitosis.

D = False This cell, which is almost certainly a B lymphocyte, is in **metaphase**. The nuclear envelope has disintegrated and the chromosomes, which have already been replicated, are lined up at the equator of the cell. The next step (**anaphase**) is that **chromosome microtubules** will pull apart the pairs of **chromatids** so that one of each pair migrates to the opposite poles of the cell, giving rise to two identical daughter cells.

E = True The cell marked **Z** is a macrophage that has phagocytosed the nuclear and cytoplasmic debris of apoptotic lymphocytes. These macrophages are plentiful in the germinal centres of active lymphoid follicles where apoptosis is common and are often called **tingible body macrophages**.

A = False This is **respiratory epithelium**, which lines the respiratory tract. The urinary tract (renal pelves, ureters, bladder and part of the urethra) is lined by **transitional epithelium**.

B = False Respiratory epithelium is a **pseudostratified ciliated columnar epithelium**. The cell nuclei are at different levels in the cells, giving the epithelium a stratified appearance. However, all the cells rest on the basement membrane and so the epithelium is not truly stratified. In contrast, stratified squamous epithelium (e.g. the epidermis of the skin) consists of layers of epithelial cells. Only the cells in the lowest (the basal) layer are in contact with the basement membrane.

C = False **Microvilli** (as exemplified by the **enterocytes** of the small intestine) are non-motile structures that greatly enlarge the surface area of absorptive cells. The surface structures in respiratory epithelium are *cilia*. These are motile and beat regularly in a coordinated fashion to carry secreted mucus and entrapped particles up the bronchial tree to the oropharynx. As a general rule of thumb, cilia can be distinguished individually in a high-power light micrograph, whereas microvilli are much smaller and only seen as a fuzzy border, e.g. the brush border of the small intestine.

D = True   *Mucus* is secreted by the *goblet cells* in the epithelium. Goblet cells are easily identified by the goblet-shaped collection of clear mucus in the upper cytoplasm. The mucus traps particles in the inspired air and carries them up the *mucociliary elevator* to clear them from the lungs. Mucus also protects the epithelial surface and helps to humidify incoming air.

E = True   The proportion of the different cell types in respiratory epithelium varies in different parts of the bronchial tree. Cell types in respiratory epithelium include tall *columnar ciliated cells*, goblet cells, *serous cells*, *stem cells*, *neuroendocrine cells* and *Clara cells*. Goblet cells are most numerous in the upper trachea but decrease in number in the distal parts of the respiratory tree. Goblet cells are absent in the terminal and respiratory bronchioles where they are replaced by Clara cells. The height of the epithelium also varies, being highest in the proximal respiratory tree and lower in the distal parts.

PAPER 2	ANSWER 2.5

A = True   *Intercalated discs* are the specialised structures found where the ends of cardiac muscle fibres abut each other. Intercalated discs hold the muscle cells together during contraction as well as providing a conduit for the very rapid spread of contractile stimuli. This is necessary for the individual muscle fibres to contract in a coordinated fashion. The need for the fibres to be strongly anchored to each other during contraction is self-evident.

B = True   Unlike skeletal and smooth muscle, cardiac muscle fibres are branched. This provides a mechanism whereby each cell is in contact with several other cells in order for contraction to be almost simultaneous.

C = True   The arrangement of the myofibrils in cardiac muscle is very similar to that of skeletal muscle, both muscle types exhibiting cross-striations if appropriately stained.

D = True   Cardiac muscle is very rich in capillaries, which are required to provide a generous supply of oxygen to muscle fibres that are contracting approximately 60–100 times per minute throughout life. The capillaries are so delicate that the capillary walls cannot be identified at this power. The presence of red blood cells in the capillary lumen, however, demonstrates the presence of a capillary.

E = False   In the past it was thought that cardiac muscle cells formed a **syncytium**, i.e. there were no boundaries between the ends of the branched muscle fibres. However, the technique of electron microscopy has demonstrated the presence of cell boundaries between the ends of the cells. These cell boundaries are characterised by intercalated discs (see A above).

A = True   This is a **simple columnar ciliated epithelium** consisting mainly of tall columnar cells with surface **cilia**. Interspersed among the columnar cells are scattered secretory cells. The secretory cells can be identified by their basal nuclei.

B = True   The surface projections are cilia, which are motile. Cilia can be differentiated from **microvilli** on light microscopy as they are much larger and can be seen individually. In contrast, microvilli are too small to see separately and consequently appear as a striated border such as in the small intestine. **Stereocilia** are much larger than cilia and appear as long thread-like surface projections. However, stereocilia are misnamed as they are actually long (non-motile) microvilli rather than motile cilia. The cilia in the Fallopian tube or oviduct move in a coordinated fashion to move the ovum towards the uterine cavity.

C = False   The cilia have a central core of pairs of doublets of **microtubules**. Nine microtubule doublets are arranged around the periphery of the cilia plus a central pair. This arrangement of microtubules is known as the **axoneme**. The peripheral microtubule doublets consist of a complete tubule that is circular in cross-section plus an incomplete C-shaped tubule attached to it. The central pair of tubules are both complete.

D = True   The **basal body** forms the base of the axoneme of each cilium. The basal body is found in the cytoplasm of the cell just deep to the cilium and consists of microtubule triplets. The inner two microtubules of the basal body are continuous with the microtubule doublet of the cilium. The central pair of microtubules of the cilium is not found in the basal body. The basal body is very similar in structure to a **centriole**.

E = True   The protein **dynein** makes up the **dynein arms**, which extend from the inner complete microtubule of each doublet. The dynein arms have ATP-ase activity and are important in the movement of the microtubule doublets.

A = False   This structure is a sensory receptor known as a **Pacinian corpuscle**. **Meissner's corpuscles** are found in the dermal papillae where they act as sensory receptors for light, discriminatory touch. They are therefore most prominent in areas such as the fingertips, eyelids, lips, etc. Meissner's corpuscles are not easily identified with routine H & E stains (or Masson's as in this case) but can be highlighted using heavy metal impregnation techniques.

B = False   The Pacinian corpuscle consists of flattened cells, which are probably modified **Schwann cells**, arranged in concentric layers rather like an onion. The outer fibrous capsule is equivalent to the onion skin. In the centre of the corpuscle there is a single non-myelinated sensory nerve fibre which does not become myelinated until it leaves the corpuscle.

C = True   Pacinian corpuscles are found in the deep part of the dermis, as well as in ligaments, joint capsules and deep soft tissue. In this case some bone can be seen in the lower portion of the micrograph.

D = False   **Merkel cells** are scattered sparsely in the basal layer of the epidermis. These cells have structures similar to synaptic vesicles in their cytoplasm. Merkel cells are closely associated with fine free sensory nerve endings in the upper dermis, and the cells and nerve endings together act as sensory receptors for touch sensation.

E = True   Pacinian corpuscles act as sensory receptors for pressure, vibration and tension. Pressure on the Pacinian corpuscle deforms its structure and by some means as yet unknown this deformity is converted into a nerve impulse. Other receptors serving similar sensory functions are **Ruffini corpuscles** in the soles of the feet and **Krause end bulbs** in the oropharynx and conjunctiva.

A = False   This cell is an **osteoclast**. These cells belong to the macrophage–monocyte lineage. Osteoclasts are responsible for resorption of bone and are found in depressions of the bone surface known as **Howship's lacunae**. Osteoclasts secrete a number of organic acids that are able to dissolve the mineral part of the bone matrix. The organic elements of the matrix are then broken up by lysosomal enzymes, which are also released by the osteoclasts. A layer of uninucleate **osteoblasts** can be seen at the margin of the bone. The other multinucleate cells which are normally found in bone are **megakaryocytes**. In practice, it is easy to distinguish the two cell types simply on the basis of their position. Osteoclasts are found in Howship's lacunae on the bone surface, while megakaryocytes are found scattered through the haemopoietic cells in the marrow spaces.

B = True   Osteoclasts are more prominent during bone healing, but are occasionally found in normal bone. During bone healing after a fracture for instance, osteoclasts are responsible for resorption of **woven bone** so that it may be replaced by **compact bone**. However, bone remodelling occurs continuously throughout life according to changes in weight bearing and use.

C = True   **Osteocytes** are found in small spaces or **lacunae** within the bone matrix. These cells are derived from osteoblasts, which become trapped in the forming bone during the laying down of new bone matrix. Although often described as inactive cells, osteocytes are important in nutrition and maintenance of the bone matrix, their fine cytoplasmic processes radiating through the canaliculi to communicate with adjacent osteocytes. In necrotic bone, the absence of osteocytes within the lacunae is an easily identifiable feature.

D = False **Parathyroid hormone** (PTH) acts to increase serum calcium levels. The bones are the major storehouse of calcium in the body and PTH acts to increase circulating calcium levels by stimulating osteoclasts to release calcium from bone.

E = True   Bone formation is a two-step process. The osteoblasts secrete both the bone matrix (**osteoid**) composed of collagen, and **matrix vesicles**. The matrix vesicles act as a focus for deposition of calcium and phosphate ions, which occurs progressively in the osteoid until it becomes fully mineralised.

PAPER 2	ANSWER 2.9

A = True   The medulla of the lymph node is made up of **medullary cords** and **medullary sinuses**. The cords are packed with cells, while the sinuses contain efferent lymph and fewer cells draining towards the **efferent lymphatic** at the hilum of the node.

B = True   Afferent lymph enters the node via multiple **afferent lymphatics**, which pierce the lymph node capsule and empty their contents into the **subcapsular sinus**. The sinus therefore contains lymphocytes, antigen-presenting cells such as **sinus macrophages** and **Langerhans cells** from the skin (known as **veiled cells** in this context). The antigen-presenting cells contain phagocytosed antigen, which they present to lymphocytes in the **cortex** of the node. The antigen is brought to the node from peripheral sites by antigen-presenting cells in order to stimulate an immune response.

C = True   The medullary sinuses contain large numbers of T lymphocytes
             as well as B lymphocytes, macrophages and plasma cells. Some
             of these lymphocytes have become activated by antigen while
             resident in the lymph node and will pass into the general
             circulation. These cells will migrate to the site where the antigen
             is to be found (e.g. a skin infection). Other lymphocytes, which
             have not been activated in the lymph node, will continue
             circulating through the nodes until they meet a suitable antigen.
             Plasma cells and **antibody**, the products of B cell activation,
             also leave the node in the efferent lymph.

D = True   This is a **secondary lymphoid follicle** (several of which are seen
             in this micrograph) consisting of a pale-staining **germinal centre**
             surrounded by a darker asymmetrical **mantle zone**. The germinal
             centre consists of mainly B lymphocytes which are undergoing
             antigenic stimulation and clonal expansion. The mantle zone
             consists of small mature B lymphocytes similar to those seen in a
             primary follicle. Primary follicles consist of small mature B
             lymphocytes. **Follicular dendritic cells**, T helper cells and
             macrophages are also found in both types of follicle.

E = True   The medullary cords are packed with **plasma cells**, the
             differentiated form of B lymphocytes. Some of these cells leave
             the node after activation, clonal expansion and differentiation,
             migrating to the site of antigen attack. Other plasma cells remain
             in the medullary cords, producing antibody that enters the general
             circulation via the efferent lymph.

PAPER 2   ANSWER 2.10

A = False   This is the **visceral pleura**. The **parietal pleura** lines the chest
             wall, whereas the visceral pleura covers the surface of the lung.
             The visceral pleura consists of a surface layer of **mesothelial
             cells** with underlying collagenous supporting tissue. The
             supporting tissue is continuous with the supporting tissue of the
             lung and with the interlobular septa. Similarly, the parietal pleura
             consists of a layer of mesothelial cells with underlying supporting
             tissue which in this case is continuous with the chest wall
             supporting tissues.

B = False   In vivo the visceral pleura is closely apposed to the surface of the
             parietal pleura, with the two layers of mesothelium separated only
             by a thin layer of pleural fluid. This fluid has a high surface
             tension so that during inspiration, when the rib cage expands, the
             visceral pleura and therefore the underlying lung are pulled along
             with the ribs, causing the lung to expand also. When air enters
             the potential pleural space, e.g. when the lung is punctured, this
             gives rise to the condition known as **pneumothorax**, a potentially
             life-threatening condition.

C = True Mesothelial cells have long surface **microvilli**, one of the major features used to identify them ultrastructurally. These cells vary in shape from flattened cuboidal to columnar, depending on the degree of expansion of the underlying lung. Like other epithelial cells, mesothelial cells rest on a basement membrane and contain **cytokeratin** (prekeratin) intermediate filaments.

D = False The flow of lymph from the pleura is from the **superficial lymph vascular plexus** to the **deep lymph vascular plexus**. Lymph then flows along the septal lymphatics to the hilar lymph nodes and thence to the **thoracic duct**.

E = True The lungs expand and contract with every breath. Elastic recoil of the lungs and pleura is important in forcing the air from the lungs during expiration. Thus, both the lung parenchyma and the pleura contain large amounts of elastin fibres.

PAPER 2   ANSWER 2.11

A = False This structure is an **epithelial crypt**. These are infoldings of the surface epithelium that dip into the **lingual tonsil**. The crypts are all in continuity with the surface although this may not be apparent depending on the plane of section. These epithelial crypts probably assist in trapping antigenic material for sampling by the underlying lymphoid tissue.

B = False **Taste buds** are found in the anterior two-thirds of the tongue. The majority are embedded in the epithelium lining the sides of the **circumvallate papillae**, dome-shaped papillae which form a V-shaped line at the junction of the anterior two-thirds with the posterior one-third. The stratified squamous epithelium of the lingual tonsil characteristically contains large numbers of lymphocytes, which are thought to sample antigen at the epithelial surface.

C = True The lingual tonsil, which is illustrated here, forms part of the collection of lymphoid structures known as **Waldeyer's ring**. The other components of Waldeyer's ring are the **palatine tonsils** and the **adenoids**. These structures are thought to form a defensive ring around the oropharynx.

D = True The lymphoid tissue of the lingual tonsil has the same general architecture as organised lymphoid tissue in other parts of the gastrointestinal tract (**gut-associated lymphoid tissue, GALT**) and indeed in lymph nodes. Lymphocytes in these tissues form aggregates known as **follicles** interspersed with **interfollicular areas** (see E below).

E = False The pale central area of this lymphoid follicle is known as the **germinal centre**. The germinal centre consists mainly of B lymphocytes, which are undergoing activation and maturation. Other cell types within the germinal centre include *helper T lymphocytes*, *follicular dendritic cells* and *tingible body macrophages*. The germinal centre is surrounded by a *mantle zone* of small inactive B lymphocytes. Together the germinal centre and mantle zone constitute a *secondary lymphoid follicle*. *Primary lymphoid follicles* consist mainly of small B cells of the type found in the mantle zone and are without a germinal centre. These follicles are inactive. The interfollicular zones, as in lymph nodes, are populated predominantly by T lymphocytes.

A = True   The columnar cells (*enterocytes*), which line the entire small intestine, have numerous *microvilli* on their luminal surface (up to 3000/cell). This feature greatly increases the surface area available for digestion and absorption of nutrients from the lumen of the small bowel. Enzymes embedded in the plasma membrane of the microvilli help to digest the food substances into small molecules, which can be transported into the cells.

B = False   *Brunner's glands*, which secrete alkaline mucus, are found only in the sub mucosa of the duodenum and are absent from the jejunum and ileum. Brunner's glands are coiled branched tubular glands with pale-staining epithelial cells. The alkali produced by these glands helps to neutralise the acid entering the duodenum from the stomach. The bulk of the Brunner's glands are situated in the submucosa but sometimes a small portion of the gland can be identified in the lamina propria.

C = True   *Paneth cells* are found clustered at the bases of the *crypts of Lieberkühn*. At this magnification the orange-red cytoplasmic granules of an occasional Paneth cell can just be seen at the base of the crypts. In Paneth cells the granules are found in the supranuclear position. In contrast, the *neuroendocrine cells* also found at the crypt bases have subnuclear reddish granules. The granules of Paneth cells contain *defensins*, which are antimicrobial peptides, as well as *lysozyme* and *phospholipase A*.

D = False   The lamina propria in the cores of the villi contains a central *lacteal*. The lacteals, the smallest branches of the lymph vascular system, are the major route for absorption of lipids from the lumen of the small intestine. Triglycerides are formed into chylomicrons in the enterocytes and then pass out of the cell, through the basement membrane and into the lacteals. The lacteals drain into larger lymphatic vessels and eventually into the *thoracic duct*.

E = True   Throughout the small and large intestine, lymphocytes are found within the epithelium of the mucosa. These **intraepithelial lymphocytes** are almost all T cells. These cells help to protect the gastrointestinal tract from invading microorganisms in conjunction with the other lymphoid cells found in lymphoid aggregates in the bowel wall and scattered through the lamina propria.

A = False **X** is a **terminal portal venule**, which is a branch of the **hepatic portal vein**. It is recognisable within the **portal tract** by its wide diameter and relatively thin wall relative to the artery and the bile ductule. The blood vessels are lined by flattened endothelium, whereas the bile ductule is lined by a simple cuboidal epithelium. The blood flows from the hepatic vein and its branches into terminal portal venules and thence to the **hepatic sinusoids**.

B = False **Y** is a terminal branch of the **hepatic artery**, which also empties into the hepatic sinusoids. It is easily recognised by its relatively thick wall of smooth muscle relative to the diameter of the lumen. In the portal tracts, the artery is approximately the same diameter as the bile ductule.

C = True   The bile ductule is lined by a cuboidal epithelium. The bile ductule, the terminal portal venule and the terminal branch of the hepatic artery make up the **portal triad** and run in the fibrous **portal tract**.

D = True   The sinusoids are blood-filled spaces between the plates of hepatocytes. The sinusoids are lined by a discontinuous layer of endothelium as well as **Kupffer cells**, neither of which are identifiable at this magnification. Kupffer cells are part of the macrophage–monocyte lineage, derived from precursor cells in the bone marrow. Like many of the cells of this lineage, Kupffer cells are able to phagocytose particles of foreign material in the blood.

E = False The classic lobule of liver architecture has a **terminal hepatic venule** at its centre and approximately six portal tracts arranged roughly around its periphery. However, a more modern and increasingly favoured unit of liver architecture is the **acinus**, which is centred on the portal tract.

A = False This micrograph shows **renal cortex**, the outer portion of the kidney. The cortex consists of **renal corpuscles** (see below) surrounded by closely packed tubules. The cortex in the adult is continuous with no division into lobes or lobules. During the development of the kidney in fetal life, the kidney is divided into lobes but these have disappeared long before adulthood. The cortex is continuous with the inner part of the kidney, the **medulla**, and is surrounded on its outer surface by a dense fibrous capsule.

B = True **Medullary rays** course through the cortex to the medulla. They consist of **collecting tubules** and **ducts** that carry the urine from the outer and mid cortex to the medulla. The collecting tubules progressively merge to form the larger **ducts of Bellini** in the **renal papilla**.

C = True The **renal corpuscle** is made up of the **glomerulus** plus **Bowman's capsule**. Between the two is **Bowman's space**, normally filled by the ultrafiltrate of plasma formed by the glomerulus and seen here as a clear space. The plasma ultrafiltrate leaves Bowman's space to enter the renal tubule where it is converted into urine.

D = False The cortex between the renal corpuscles is packed with renal tubules but the bulk of the tissue is made up of **proximal convoluted tubules** (**PCT**) as they are longer than **distal convoluted tubules** (**DCT**). The PCT in their tortuous course therefore occupy a larger volume than the DCT. The tubules convert the ultrafiltrate of plasma produced by the glomeruli into urine by selective reabsorption of some substances, such as glucose and sodium, and selective secretion of others, such as hydrogen ions and water.

E = False This is a **cortical radial vein**, which can be identified as a vein by its wide-diameter lumen in comparison to its relatively thin wall. The **cortical radial arteries** and their veins run radially from the junction of the cortex and medulla to the outer cortex. They are branches of the **arcuate arteries** and **veins** that run in an arch-like fashion along the corticomedullary junction. The arcuate arteries and veins are in turn branches of the **interlobar arteries** and **veins**, which again take a radial course through the medulla and originate from the major branches of the **renal artery** and **vein** at the **hilum** of the kidney.

PAPER 2	ANSWER 2.15

A = True **X** marks the **adrenal medulla**, which secretes the catecholamine hormones **adrenaline** (**epinephrine**) and **noradrenaline** (**norepinephrine**). The cells of the adrenal medulla contain adrenaline and noradrenaline in membrane-bound dense core granules in the cytoplasm. The hormones are released in response to stimulation by preganglionic neurones of the sympathetic nervous system. These cells therefore function essentially as postganglionic nerve cells. The hormones noradrenaline and adrenaline cause the 'flight or fight' response well known to all junior doctors who have ever been part of the cardiac arrest team.

B = False **Y** marks the **central vein** of the medulla, which receives blood from both medulla and **cortex** of the adrenal gland. This vessel can be recognised as a vein because of its wide diameter in relation to the thickness of its wall. The **long cortical arteries** arise in the **subcapsular plexus** and course through the cortex to supply the medulla. The **short cortical arteries** also arise in the subcapsular plexus and supply the cortex.

C = False The zone identified by **Z** is the **zona glomerulosa**, the outermost layer of the cortex. The middle layer is the **zona fasciculata** and the innermost layer the **zona reticularis**. In the zona glomerulosa the endocrine cells are arranged in small clusters. In the fasciculata, the cells are arranged in cords at right angles to the capsule. The reticular layer is composed of smaller more irregular cords of cells.

D = True The zona glomerulosa is the main site of production of **mineralocorticoids**, mainly **aldosterone**. This hormone, in conjunction with the renin–angiotensin system, acts to regulate systemic blood pressure. In contrast, the zonae fasciculata and reticularis produce **glucocorticoids**, principally **cortisol**, and small amounts of **sex hormones**.

E = True This is the zona fasciculata of the adrenal cortex. The cells of all three layers of the adrenal cortex contain large amounts of **smooth endoplasmic reticulum** (sER), the site of steroid hormone production. Lipid droplets, the substrate for hormone synthesis, are also found in these cells but are most prominent in the zona fasciculata. The cells of the zona fasciculata have copious pale cytoplasm owing to their content of lipid droplets.

PAPER 2	ANSWER 2.16

A = False This is a high-power micrograph of **anterior pituitary** tissue. The anterior pituitary is made up of clusters and branching cords of epithelial cells derived from a structure arising in the embryonic oral cavity known as **Rathke's pouch**. The **posterior pituitary** consists of modified neurones, the cell bodies of which are found in the **hypothalamus. Pituicytes**, which resemble **glial cells** of the central nervous system, are also found in the posterior pituitary.

B = True In common with most other endocrine glands, the anterior pituitary has an extensive network of **fenestrated capillaries**, which facilitate entry of hormones into the general circulation. In fenestrated capillaries the cytoplasm of the endothelial cells lining the capillary forms multiple small pores which can be seen by electron microscopy. The pores may be bridged by a thin diaphragm. In this micrograph there are many capillaries, which can usually be identified by their content of blood cells. In this particular case the blood cells have largely been washed out during preparation and only an occasional erythrocyte can be seen within the capillaries. Endocrine glands, in contrast to exocrine glands, have no ducts.

C = True   The anterior pituitary secretes a wide range of hormones including **growth hormone**, **prolactin**, **adrenocorticotrophin**, **thyrotrophin**, **luteinising hormone** and **follicle stimulating hormone**. The secretory products are packaged into **secretory granules** that can be seen by electron microscopy. These secretory granules vary in size, position and number according to the type of hormone produced by a particular cell, and the different cell types can be recognised by the characteristics of their granules. As a general rule one cell secretes one type of hormone. Electron microscopy is too time-consuming for general diagnostic purposes, and identification of different cell types is generally carried out using immunohistochemical techniques. A common example would be to confirm the presence of a **pituitary adenoma**, which is generally composed of a single cell type as opposed to the mixture of cell types found in normal pituitary.

D = False   Although the individual cell types are scattered unevenly throughout the gland, most cell clusters contain a mixture of different cell types with different secretory products.

E = False   **Vasopressin** or **antidiuretic hormone** (**ADH**) is the product of the posterior pituitary. ADH is synthesised by the neurone cell bodies of the hypothalamus (specifically in the **supraoptic nucleus**). The ADH passes along the axons in the **pituitary stalk** and is stored in the ends of the axons, which are expanded. Release of ADH occurs in response to nerve impulses along the axons.

PAPER 2	ANSWER 2.17

A = False   This is a **seminiferous tubule**. The parenchyma of the testis is made up of seminiferous tubules separated by a delicate interstitium. The seminiferous tubules are the site of production of **spermatozoa**. The **rete testis** (not seen in this micrograph) is a complex of channels found in the **mediastinum testis**. The spermatozoa formed in the seminiferous tubules pass into the rete testis and from there via the **ductuli efferentes** into the **epididymis** (see **E** below). The rete testis allows mixing of spermatozoa, a process assisted by contraction of myoid cells found in the collagenous supporting tissue of the mediastinum testis. The simple cuboidal epithelium of the rete also functions to reabsorb potassium and protein from the seminal fluid.

B = True   The **tunica albuginea**, the dense fibrous capsule of the testis, is not seen in this micrograph. The **interlobular septa** of the testis are continuous with the tunica albuginea and divide the testis into lobules, each containing up to four seminiferous tubules. The outer layer of the tunica albuginea consists of dense collagenous tissue containing fibroblasts and myofibroblasts. The deeper layer of the tunica albuginea is composed of looser collagenous tissue containing blood vessels and lymphatics, known as the **tunica vasculosa**. On the surface of the tunica albuginea is a single layer of mesothelium, known as the **visceral tunica vaginalis**. The **parietal tunica vaginalis** lines the scrotum.

C = True   The lining of the seminiferous tubules is composed of two cell types, the **spermatogenic series** and **Sertoli cells**. Sertoli cells are large cells that rest on the basement membrane of the seminiferous tubule and extend to the lumen. They have branched cytoplasm that ramifies between the spermatogenic cells forming a network within which the spermatogenic cells divide and develop. In particular, they divide the seminiferous tubule lining into **basal** and **adluminal compartments**. Sertoli cells act as support cells for the spermatogenic cells and secrete a variety of regulatory factors.

D = False   The final stage of the maturation of spermatozoa, the development of motility, occurs in the epididymis (see below).

E = True   The **epididymis** is a coiled tube found along the posterior margin of the testis. In cross-section as seen here it appears as a mass of circular spaces, lined by epithelium and embedded in a fibrous stroma. The epididymis is the site of storage and final maturation of spermatozoa. Note the first part of the **vas deferens** near the top of the micrograph.

A = False   The **lacuna system** (**X**) is filled with maternal blood in vivo. Fetal blood can be seen in this micrograph in the delicate capillaries in the centre of the **chorionic villi**. Exchange of oxygen and nutrients occurs across the intervening tissue of the villus.

B = True   The **chorionic villi** make up the parenchyma of the placenta. The villi are formed by branching of the primary chorionic villi to form secondary and tertiary chorionic villi. The villi in this micrograph are tertiary villi with a core of **mesenchyme** and central small blood vessels.

C = False   The cells on the surface of the chorionic villi consist of a deep layer of **cytotrophoblast** and a superficial layer of **syncytiotrophoblast**, so called because the cells form a syncytium, appearing as multinucleate cells on the surface of the villi. In later pregnancy the cytotrophoblast layer partly disappears leaving a single layer of syncytiotrophoblast on the surface.

D = True   During the development of the placenta, chorionic villi form by budding of solid cores of **intermediate trophoblast**. This gives a complex structure with multiple generations of branches which present an enormous surface area to the maternal blood in the lacuna system for gas and nutrient exchange.

E = True   The core of the chorionic villus consists of mesenchymal cells in a myxoid matrix. The mesenchyme supports the fetal capillaries, which in this first trimester placenta are centrally placed in the villi. In later pregnancy, as the oxygen and nutrient requirements of the growing fetus increase, the capillaries are larger and more peripherally placed to reduce the tissue barrier between maternal and fetal blood.

PAPER 2	ANSWER 2.19

A = True   The bulk of the **cornea** consists of layers or **laminae** of dense collagenous tissue. Cells are scanty but occasional **fibroblasts**, which produce the collagen, are found. This is the **substantia propria** or stroma of the cornea.

B = False   This structure is **Descemet's membrane**. This is a thick membrane of elastic fibres and collagen that lines the inner surface of the cornea. **Bowman's membrane** is the specialised layer of the corneal stroma that lies between the surface epithelium and the substantia propria. Thus the substantia propria is bounded anteriorly by Bowman's membrane and posteriorly by Descemet's membrane.

C = True   The single layer of squamous cells lining the posterior surface of the cornea is thought to be specialised endothelium. These cells remove fluid from the cornea (which is avascular) and pump it into the **anterior chamber** of the eye.

D = False   The surface epithelium of the cornea is a **non-keratinised stratified squamous epithelium. Transitional epithelium** is only found in the urogenital system. This surface epithelium produces no lubricating fluid but is lubricated by the secretions of the **lacrimal glands** (tears) and conjunctiva, thus ensuring that the eyelids can move without friction over the surface of the eye.

E = True   The outer layer of the globe is the **corneoscleral layer**. The posterior two-thirds is the **sclera**, which consists of dense collagenous tissue and gives structural support to the eye. The anterior portion of this layer is the transparent cornea, which as well as forming the anterior wall of the eye, is part of the optical system, focusing light on the **retina**. The cornea makes up approximately one-sixth of the outer layer of the eye.

A = True   This is the **follicular antrum** of this ovarian follicle (**Graafian follicle**). The follicular antrum begins to appear in the **secondary follicle** as small fluid-filled spaces, which eventually coalesce to make a single space. The **oocyte** is surrounded by layers of **granulosa cells** in the **cumulus oophorus** that is seen protruding into the follicular antrum.

B = False   The area marked **Y** is composed of granulosa cells and is called the **zona granulosa**. The follicular cells of the **primordial follicle** divide by mitosis to form a thick border of granulosa cells around the oocyte of the **primary follicle**. As the follicle continues to mature, fluid collects between the granulosa cells to coalesce into the follicular antrum of the Graafian follicle. The granulosa cells are a major part of the **corpus luteum** after ovulation and are responsible for the secretion of progesterone.

C = True   The **zona pellucida** is a thick layer made up of acid proteoglycans and glycoprotein, separating the zona granulosa from the oocyte.

D = True   The primordial follicle develops through three stages before ovulation. These are in order: primary follicle, secondary follicle and Graafian follicle. Just before ovulation the granulosa cell bridges that attach the oocyte to the wall of the follicle break down so that the oocyte floats free in the follicle surrounded by the zona pellucida and a **corona radiata** of granulosa cells. These three components make up the mature **ovum**, which is ejected from the ovary at the time of ovulation.

E = False   This is the **theca interna**, composed of modified ovarian **stromal cells**. In this example the theca interna is easily distinguished. The theca interna cells are more rounded than typical stromal cells and contain lipid and plentiful smooth endoplasmic reticulum in their cytoplasm. These cells secrete oestrogen and its precursors and some progestagens. The theca interna is surrounded by the **theca externa** of spindle-shaped cells, which blend with the surrounding stroma.

A = False   The structure labelled **X** is a **focal density**. There are several of these visible in these smooth muscle cells. Focal densities act as anchoring points for the contractile filaments in the cytoplasm of the smooth muscle cell. **Desmin**, the intermediate filament that is an important component of the **cytoskeleton**, is also attached to the focal densities. Thus when the filaments contract the cell changes shape. **Anchoring densities** are similar structures on the plasma membrane of the cell.

B = True This is part of a smooth muscle cell nucleus. Smooth muscle cell nuclei are centrally placed in the cell in contrast to skeletal muscle where the nuclei are found in the periphery of the cell. Note also the random arrangement of mitochondria in the cell in contrast to the highly ordered arrangement of mitochondria in skeletal muscle.

C = True *Actin* and *myosin filaments* can be seen occupying most of the cytoplasm of these smooth muscle cells. In contrast to skeletal muscle, the contractile filaments are arranged in a seemingly haphazard pattern. However, as mentioned above, the filaments are anchored in such a way that shortening of the contractile filaments changes the shape of the cells.

D = True Part of a small nerve bundle is included in this field. Note the multiple nerve axons cut in various planes of section. These are unmyelinated nerve fibres and many of the nerves probably belong to the autonomic nervous system.

E = True Smooth muscle cells communicate with each other via *gap* or *nexus junctions*, which allow the rapid transmission of a nerve stimulus through adjacent muscle cells. In this way contraction of adjacent cells can be synchronised. This micrograph is of too low magnification to allow identification of gap junctions.

PAPER 2	ANSWER 2.22

A = False This is an *eosinophil*, easily recognised by its *specific granules*. The granules are membrane-bound and of fairly uniform size. The key feature of the granules is the elongated *crystalloid* structure found within them. In this eosinophil, which used to belong to rat, the granules are more electron-dense (darker) than the surrounding material. In humans the reverse is true, with less electron-dense granules surrounded by denser material.

B = True Eosinophils generally have a bilobed nucleus. This cell probably also has a bilobed nucleus but it is not visible in the plane of section. The nucleus of neutrophils is polylobated, hence the name *polymorphonuclear neutrophil*, while the nucleus of the other granulocyte, the *basophil*, is bilobed like that of the eosinophil. Basophils and eosinophils can be differentiated from each other at the light microscopic level by the different colour of the granules: basophils have basophilic (blue) granules, whereas eosinophils have eosinophilic (pink) granules. By electron microscopy, eosinophils can be identified by the distinctive crystalloids in the cytoplasmic granules. Basophils have much greater numbers of granules.

C = False *Immunoglobulins* are secreted by plasma cells, which are derived from lymphocytes. The secretory products of eosinophils, which are stored in the granules, include *major basic protein*, *histaminase*, hydrolytic lysosomal enzymes and *peroxidase*.

D = True   Eosinophils have surface receptors for IgE. It is likely that IgE bound to the surface of eosinophils works together with the secretory products of eosinophils to destroy parasites. Eosinophils are also found within the tissue in certain *hypersensitivity* (*allergic*) *reactions*. For instance, in allergic type *nasal polyps*, eosinophils are often prominent.

E = True   Eosinophils, as mentioned above, are important in the defence against parasites. Eosinophils are attracted to the site of parasitic infection, for instance schistosomes in the bladder, by chemotactic factors. As the parasites are too large to be phagocytosed by the eosinophil, the eosinophils are thought to release their granule contents in the vicinity of the parasite, thus damaging the parasite.

PAPER 2	ANSWER 2.23

A = True   **X** marks the *alveolar space* or air space. In life this area would be filled with air. It is separated from the capillary, which occupies most of the field in this micrograph, by the combined alveolar and capillary wall.

B = False   The structure marked **Y** is the cytoplasm of a *type I pneumocyte*. The alveolar spaces are separated from the capillaries by a thin layer of type I pneumocyte cytoplasm, endothelial cell cytoplasm and between the two a fused basement membrane. This structure forms the main barrier for diffusion of gases between the inspired air and the capillaries. The pneumocyte cytoplasm is on the air side of this barrier, while the endothelial cell cytoplasm is on the capillary side.

C = False   The cell marked **Z** is a *reticulocyte*. The lumen of the capillary can be identified as in many other tissues by its content of blood cells. In this field, as well as a reticulocyte, there is part of a mature erythrocyte in the lower left of the field. The mature erythrocyte has characteristic dumbbell shape. Note that the cytoplasm of the erythrocyte is homogeneous. In contrast the cytoplasm of the reticulocyte contains a few mitochondria, some profiles of smooth endoplasmic reticulum and two fragments of nuclear material seen in approximately the centre of the cell. In the maturation of erythrocytes, the reticulocyte is the stage immediately before the formation of mature erythrocytes. The reticulocyte must extrude nuclear fragments and other organelles to become an erythrocyte.

D = False   **W** marks the fused basement membrane of the type I pneumocyte and the endothelial cell. *Type II pneumocytes* are found in the angles between adjacent alveolae and in that area make some contribution to the production of the basement membrane. However, in the area seen in this micrograph, the basement membrane is produced by both the endothelial cells and the type I pneumocyte.

E = False   **Y** as mentioned above is the cytoplasm of a type I pneumocyte. *Lamellar bodies* are characteristic of type II pneumocytes. These are found at the angles between adjacent alveolae and bulge into the air space in this area. Lamellar bodies are membrane-bound organelles composed mainly of phospholipids and have a layered structure. These are not found in type I pneumocytes. The lamellae store some of the components of surfactant, which reduces surface tension on the surface of the alveolae and prevents adherence between the alveolar walls when they come into contact. Very premature infants who are not yet able to secrete surfactant are unable to inflate their alveolae and maintain the inflation. These infants often suffer from *infant respiratory distress syndrome*, also known as *hyaline membrane disease*.

A = True   *Microtubules* are plentiful in the axons of nerves. When seen in longitudinal section as here, they appear as long hollow tubes with a diameter of 24 nm. In transverse section they are small hollow circles. Microtubules are made up of two types of subunit, *alpha* and *beta tubulin*. These polymerise to form the tubule, with 13 subunits making one complete circle. Microtubules are important in the movement of materials within the cell. For instance, microtubules move the separated chromatids to the opposite poles of the dividing cell. Microtubules are closely associated within the cell with the *centriole*, sometimes known as the *microtubule organising centre*.

B = False   The *myelin sheath* is easily recognised by its layered structure with alternating pale and dark lines. **Y** marks the cytoplasm of a *Schwann cell*, which is wrapped around this unmyelinated nerve fibre. The separate plasma membranes of the nerve axon and Schwann cell can best be identified at the upper left corner of this micrograph. Neither the nucleus of the Schwann cell nor that of the nerve is included in the micrograph.

C = True   Microtubules become longer or shorter by the addition or subtraction of subunits. For instance during cell division the *chromatids* are pulled to opposite poles of the cell by shortening of the attached microtubules (the *chromosome* or *kinetochore microtubules*). At the same time the *interpolar microtubules* add subunits to elongate, pushing apart the two halves of the cell. This is controlled by the centrioles at the opposite poles of the dividing cell. Chromosomes or cell organelles are attached to the microtubules by the proteins **dynein** and **kynesin**. Dynein is also associated with the microtubule doublets found in cilia.

D = False   The **intermediate filaments** found in Schwann cells are similar to those found in glial cells of the CNS, known as **glial fibrillary acidic protein** or **GFAP**. Peripheral nerve cells in common with other nerve cells contain **neurofilament proteins**, intermediate filaments specific for this cell type.

E = True   Intermediate filaments are easily seen in both the axon and the Schwann cell. Intermediate filaments are seen as solid lines measuring 10–15 nm in diameter. Intermediate filaments make up an important part of the **cytoskeleton** and unlike **microfilaments** and microtubules have a stable structure. As mentioned above, different classes of intermediate filament are found in different cell lineages: **cytokeratin** is characteristic of epithelial cells, neurofilament proteins are specific for nerve cells, **desmin** is the muscle intermediate filament, GFAP is found in glial cells and **vimentin** is seen in cells of mesenchymal origin.

PAPER 3

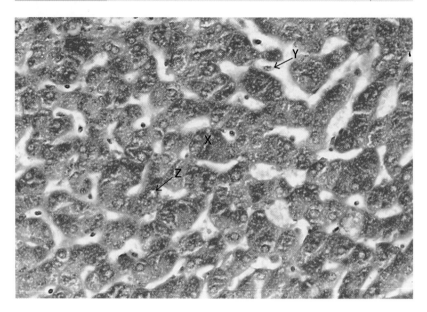

In this high-power photomicrograph of liver stained by the PAS method:

A   The bright pink granular material seen by this staining method in the cytoplasm of the hepatocytes (**X**) is mucus

B   The cell marked **Y** is a resting hepatocyte.

C   The structure marked **Z** is a large lipid droplet.

D   The cytoplasmic pink granular material in the hepatocytes is located within membrane-bound vesicles.

E   The cell marked **X** has plentiful mitochondria in the cytoplasm.

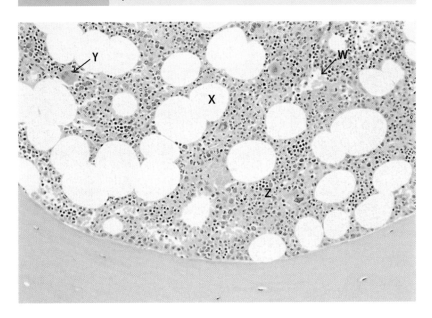

In this micrograph of normal bone marrow:

A   The cell marked **X** is an adipocyte.

B   The structure marked **Y** is a megakaryocyte.

C   **Z** marks normal haemopoietic tissue.

D   **W** indicates a small artery supplying the marrow.

E   **W** is lined by a fenestrated endothelium.

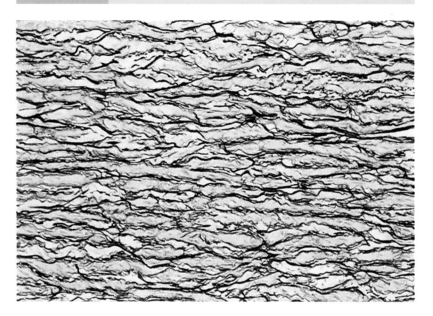

In this micrograph of the aorta stained with a special method for elastin, which stains elastin blackish-brown:

A   The elastin fibres form concentric layers in the tunica media.

B   Elastin is prominent in the epidermis as well as the dermis.

C   Elastin is composed of polymerised tropoelastin.

D   Elastin is closely associated with fibrillin in the tissues.

E   Elastin is synthesised by tissue macrophages.

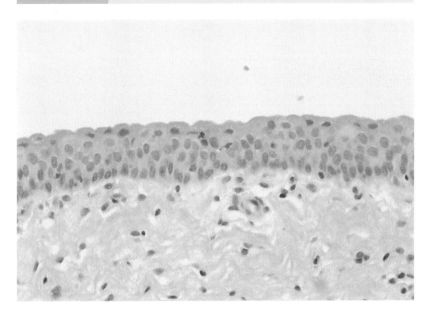

In this high-power view of the mucosa of the urinary bladder:

A   Keratinisation is seen on the surface of the epithelium.

B   The surface cells have a specialised plasma membrane.

C   Binucleate cells are common in all layers.

D   Mucus-secreting cells are scattered along the surface.

E   The epithelium is normally from two to five cell layers thick.

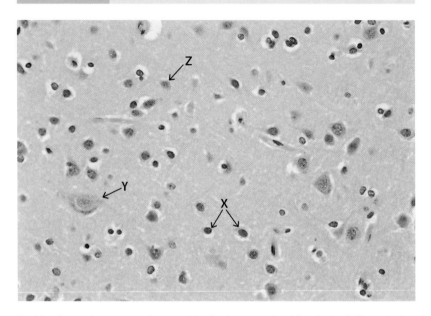

In this photomicrograph of normal brain tissue stained by the H & E method:

A The cells marked **X** are lymphocytes.

B The darker-stained area in the cytoplasm of the cell marked **Y** is composed of rough endoplasmic reticulum.

C The cell marked **Z** has multiple axons which synapse with similar cells.

D The material between cell nuclei is known as neuropil.

E The tissue was taken from the medulla of the cerebral hemispheres.

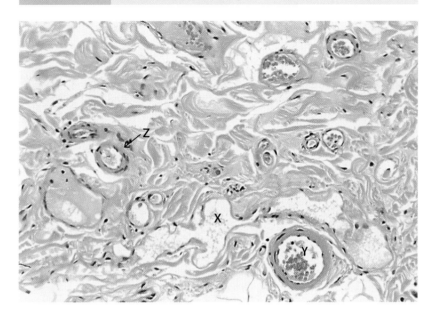

In this low-power photomicrograph of loose collagenous supporting tissue:

A The structure marked **X** is a lymphatic.

B The structure identified by **Y** is an arteriole.

C The structure identified by **Y** is lined by fenestrated endothelium.

D The structure marked **Z** is an elastic artery.

E The structure marked **X** does not contain valves.

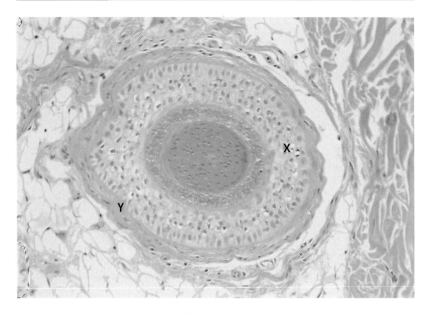

In this photomicrograph of a hair follicle:

A   The hair shaft consists of three layers.

B   The hair shaft is produced by cells found in the internal root sheath of the hair.

C   The structure marked **X** consists mainly of melanocytes.

D   The glassy membrane is marked by **Y**.

E   The shape of the hair follicle is one of the factors that determines whether the hair is straight or curly.

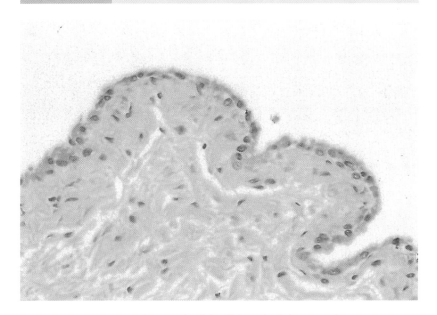

In this medium-power micrograph of the lining of a joint capsule:

A   The surface cell layers are of mesenchymal origin.

B   The surface cell layers rest on a basement membrane.

C   The surface cell layers secrete joint fluid.

D   This type of joint lining is found in the facet joints of the spinous processes of the vertebrae.

E   The tissue underlying the surface layers contains few capillaries.

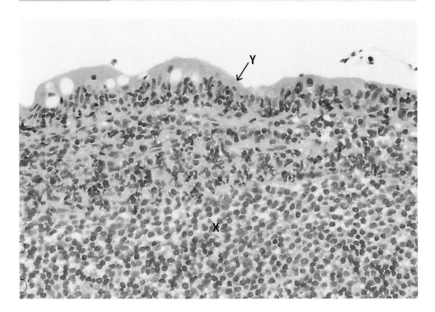

In this micrograph of the superficial part of a Peyer's patch in the ileum:

A   The cells in the area marked **X** are mainly T lymphocytes.

B   Lymphoid cells from this site migrate to skin.

C   Peyer's patches are found throughout the large and small bowel.

D   The covering epithelium (**Y**) includes M cells.

E   Peyer's patches are a major site of secretory IgA synthesis.

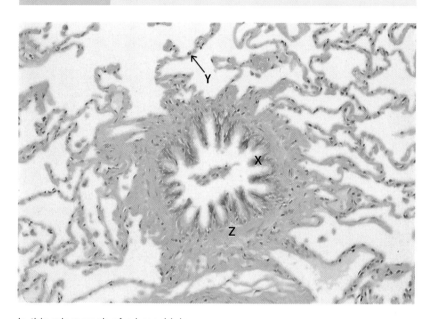

In this micrograph of a bronchiole:

A The epithelium **X** includes Kulchitsky cells.

B Neuroendocrine cells in the epithelium are characterised by plentiful cytoplasmic synaptic vesicles.

C The epithelium contains Clara cells.

D The structure marked **Y** is lined on both sides by endothelium.

E The area marked **Z** consists of smooth muscle.

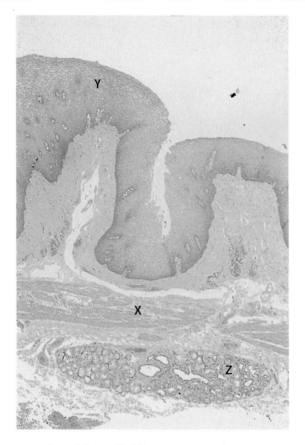

In this low-power view of the wall of the upper oesophagus:

A   The structure marked **X** contains a mixture of smooth and striated muscle.

B   The structure marked **Y** is a keratinised stratified squamous epithelium in humans.

C   The outermost layer of the oesophageal wall (not illustrated) is a layer of mesothelium.

D   Parasympathetic ganglion cells are found in clusters in the structure marked **X**.

E   The structure marked **Z** is a seromucinous gland.

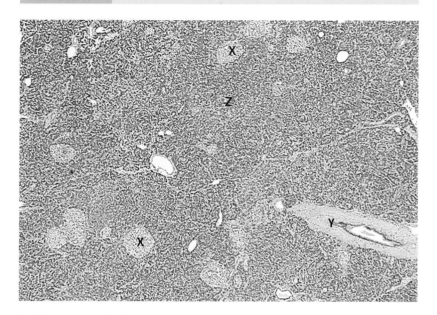

In this micrograph of pancreas:

A   The structures marked **X** are responsible for the production of glucagon.

B   The products of the structures marked **X** are excreted into the duodenum via the structure marked **Y**.

C   An electron micrograph of the cells in the area marked **Z** would show cells rich in smooth endoplasmic reticulum.

D   The structure marked **Y** drains into an intercalated duct.

E   The cells in the area marked **Z** contain zymogen granules.

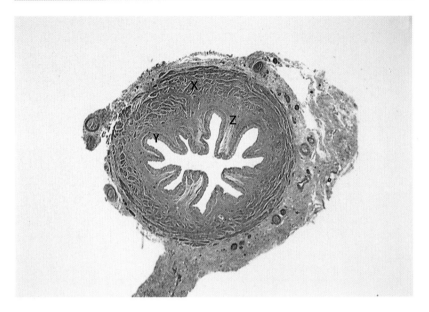

In this photomicrograph of the ureter stained with the Masson's trichrome method:

A   The structure marked **X** consists of layers of skeletal muscle.

B   The lining epithelium **Y** is the same type as the epithelium lining the bladder.

C   The layer deep to the epithelium (**Z**) carries the major blood vessels supplying the ureter.

D   The outermost layer of the ureter has a mesothelial lining similar to the peritoneum.

E   The muscle layer of the ureter undergoes regular spontaneous contraction.

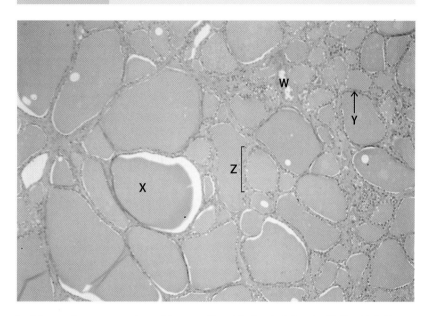

In this medium-power view of human thyroid gland stained with the H & E method:

A   The material marked **X** is the site of storage of calcitonin within the gland.

B   The cells marked **Y** may form a stratified epithelium when the gland is more active.

C   The structure marked **Z** is a follicle.

D   The capillary marked **W** has a fenestrated endothelium.

E   C cells can be easily identified.

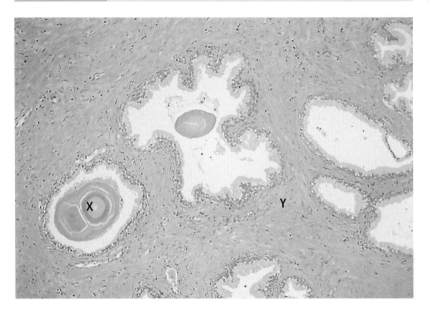

In this high-power photomicrograph of the prostate gland:

A   The structure marked **X** is a feature commonly seen in the prostates of young boys.

B   The glandular epithelium is a simple columnar epithelium.

C   Brown lipofuscin pigment can be seen within the epithelial cells.

D   The secretory product of these glands is rich in citric acid and hydrolytic enzymes.

E   The area marked **Y** is likely to contain smooth muscle fibres.

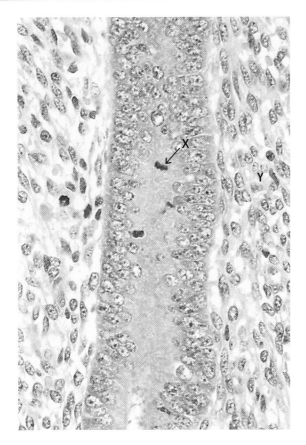

In this high-magnification micrograph of endometrium:

A   The endometrium is in the late secretory phase of the menstrual cycle.

B   The feature indicated by **X** is a subnuclear vacuole.

C   The cells in the area marked **Y** are myometrial cells.

D   The gland epithelium is a pseudostratified columnar epithelium.

E   The individual from whom this specimen was taken has already ovulated.

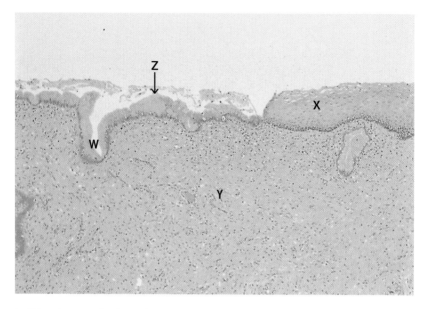

In this micrograph of cervix:

A   The epithelium marked **X** is transitional epithelium.

B   The tissue marked **Y** is made up mainly of smooth muscle.

C   The epithelium marked **Z** is a simple columnar mucus-secreting epithelium.

D   The endocervical gland marked **W** is similar to endometrial glands.

E   The 'Pap smear' is a technique for examining the epithelial cells of the cervix for precancerous changes.

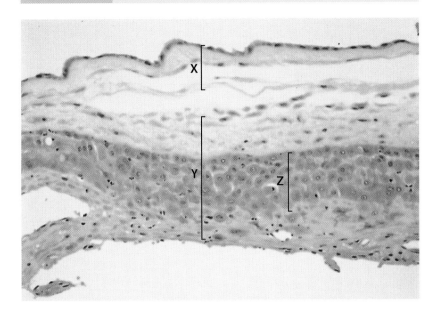

In this photomicrograph of fetal membranes:

A   **X** marks the amnion.

B   The chorion (**Y**) is composed of three layers.

C   The layer marked **Z** is derived from trophoblast.

D   The structure marked **X** consists of cells derived from the mother.

E   **X** is closest to the fetus.

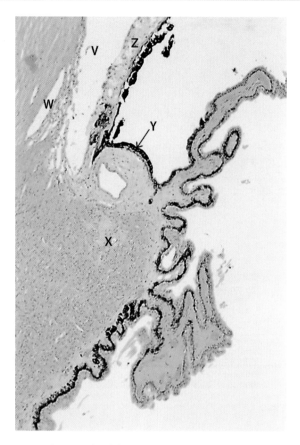

In this low-power micrograph of the eye:

A   The structure marked **X** is the ciliary body.

B   The pigmented layer marked **Y** contains rods and cones.

C   The structure marked **Z** is the iris.

D   The structure marked **W** is important in the circulation of the aqueous humor.

E   The area marked **V** is the anterior chamber.

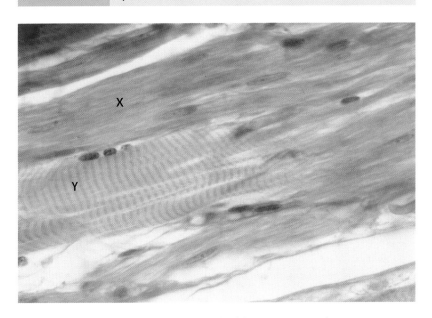

In this high-power micrograph of the wall of the upper oesophagus:

A   The muscle fibres marked **X** contain thick contractile filaments but not thin filaments.

B   The muscle fibres marked **Y** are skeletal muscle fibres.

C   The muscle fibres marked **X** have their contractile filaments anchored to focal densities.

D   The muscle fibres marked **Y** have their contractile filaments arranged in sarcomeres.

E   The arrangement of muscle fibres is similar to that seen at the ileocaecal valve.

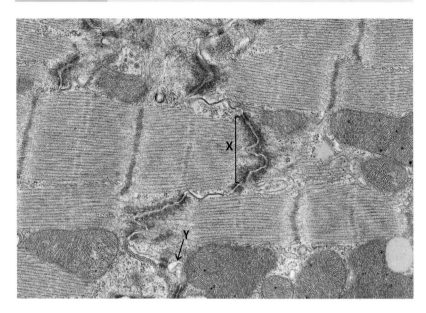

In this high-power electron micrograph of cardiac muscle:

A   The muscle fibres are joined at their blunt ends by an intercalated disc.

B   The structure marked **X** is a fascia adherens.

C   The structure marked **Y** is a mitochondrion.

D   Glycogen granules act as an energy source.

E   Each muscle cell has a separate nerve connection.

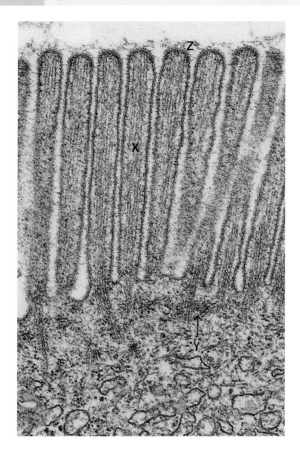

In this high-power electron micrograph of small bowel epithelium:

A   The structure marked **X** is a cilium.

B   The structure marked **X** has a core of actin filaments.

C   The structure marked **Y** is the terminal web.

D   The material marked **Z** is the glycocalyx.

E   Similar structures to **X** are found in large numbers on the luminal surface of the epithelium of the bronchi.

In the medium-power electron micrograph of lung tissue on the facing page:

A　The cell marked **X** is a type I pneumocyte.

B　The structure marked **Y** is a lamellar body.

C　The cell marked **X** is usually found within the wall of a bronchiole.

D　The structure marked **Z** is a capillary.

E　The structure marked **W** is part of the cytoplasm of a type I pneumocyte.

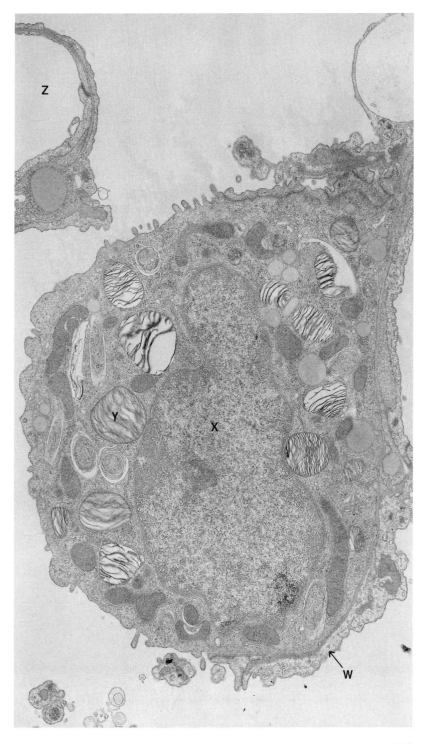

119

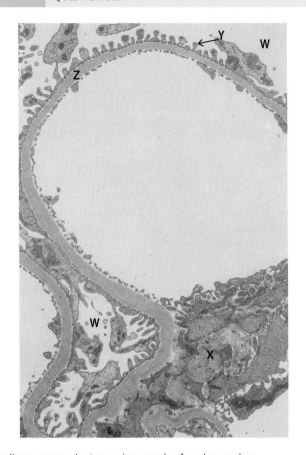

In this medium-power electron micrograph of a glomerulus:

A   The structure marked **X** contains material similar to basement membrane.

B   The structure marked **Y** is fenestrated endothelium.

C   The structure marked **Z** consists of three layers.

D   The area marked **W** would be filled with blood in vitro.

E   The area marked **X** contains cells capable of phagocytosis.

A = False   The material stained bright pink is **glycogen**, which is typically found in large amounts in the cytoplasm of **hepatocytes**. Hepatocytes do not normally produce mucus. Mucus does however, stain with this staining method. To differentiate between mucus and glycogen, which is important in some diagnostic settings (adenocarcinoma cells contain mucus as well as glycogen, while many other cell types contain glycogen but no mucus), the tissue section is pretreated with the enzyme diastase before staining. Usually two slides are stained in parallel, one treated with diastase and the other not. Diastase breaks down glycogen but not mucus. Thus the presence of PAS-positive material (bright pink) on the diastase-treated slide demonstrates the presence of mucus. Material that stains on the non-diastase-treated slides but is unstained on the treated slide is identified as glycogen. For example, if the tissue section shown in this micrograph had been pretreated with diastase before staining, there would have been no pink staining in the cytoplasm.

B = False   This is a **Kupffer cell**, which belongs to the macrophage–monocyte lineage and is one of the lining cells of the **liver sinusoids**. These cells have inconspicuous cytoplasm and smaller darker nuclei than the hepatocytes. Like other cells in this group, Kupffer cells are phagocytic and remove particulate material from the blood as it percolates through the sinusoids. The other cells found lining the liver sinusoids include **endothelial cells** and **stellate** or **Ito cells**.

C = False   This is the hepatocyte nucleus. No lipid droplets are seen in these normal hepatocytes. The presence of lipid droplets in liver cells, known as **steatosis** or **fatty liver**, is a feature of many pathological conditions including **alcoholic liver disease**. Lipid appears as clear unstained spaces in routinely processed tissue as the processing fluids dissolve out the lipid from the tissue. In order to demonstrate lipid in tissue, special preparation techniques and stains are required.

D = False   Glycogen is found as single particles (α **particles**) or groups of particles (β **particles**) in the cytoplasm. There is no encircling membrane. The particles are slightly larger than **ribosomes**. Free ribosomes and glycogen α granules can, however, be difficult to differentiate in electron micrographs by the non-expert. Glycogen is found in almost all cell types where it acts as a readily available energy store.

E = True   Mitochondria are present in fairly large numbers in hepatocytes, which are highly metabolically active cells requiring copious amounts of energy. Mitochondria do not, however, stain with the PAS method so that although they are present in the cytoplasm they do not stain strongly.

121

A = True   The bone marrow contains variable numbers of **adipocytes** (fat cells). In inactive **yellow marrow** such as that found in the shafts of the long bones of adults, the marrow consists mainly of adipose tissue with only scattered, inconspicuous **haemopoietic cells** (blood cell precursors). **Red marrow**, on the other hand, consists of approximately equal amounts of adipose tissue and haemopoietic tissue, as in this photograph. There is a gradual transition between red marrow and yellow marrow and the amount of haemopoietic tissue varies according to the requirement for production of blood cells. For instance, after a major haemorrhage, the proportion of haemopoietic cells in the marrow increases to replace the lost blood cells.

B = True   **Megakaryocytes**, the cells that give rise to platelets, are usually easily recognised in sections and smears of bone marrow. They have multisegmented nuclei and plentiful eosinophilic cytoplasm. The cell margin often appears irregular or ragged owing to the budding of platelets. Megakaryocytes should not be confused with **osteoclasts** in tissue sections. Osteoclasts are found closely apposed to the bone surface or in a small concavity (**Howship's lacuna**) on the bone surface. These multinucleate cells are members of the monocyte–macrophage lineage and are responsible for bone resorption.

C = True   Normal haemopoietic tissue contains mature blood cells of all types and their precursors in all stages of development. Plasma cells are also a normal component as well as **reticular cells** (fibroblasts) and adipocytes as mentioned above. These cells are supported by a delicate reticulin framework. At first glance (and often at second glance) bone marrow seems totally chaotic. However, the marrow is a highly organised tissue. Cells of a particular lineage tend to occur in clusters that include all stages of maturation.

D = False   **W** marks a marrow **sinusoid**. These are wide-diameter capillaries, which not only supply oxygen and nutrients to the marrow but also provide a means of entry for blood cells into the circulation. The sinusoids form an extensive three-dimensional meshwork throughout the marrow spaces.

E = False   The sinusoids are lined by a continuous endothelium which rests on a discontinuous basement membrane. The flattened elongated nuclei of the endothelial cells can be identified in higher-power micrographs. Surrounding the sinusoids is a meshwork of stellate cells known as reticular cells, which are actually a type of fibroblast. The reticular cells appear to be able to accumulate lipid in their cytoplasm and become identical to adipose cells in inactive marrow.

A = True   **Elastin** fibres form concentric layers throughout the **tunica media** of elastic arteries such as the aorta. Elastin is arranged in different patterns in different tissues. For instance the **internal** and **external elastic laminae** of muscular arteries, such as the femoral arteries, are thick layers of elastin found at the margins of the tunica media. Elastin fibres form a three-dimensional network in supporting tissue such as the dermis of the skin and are present in almost all supporting tissues in the body. Elastin is particularly prominent in organs which expand and contract such as the lungs, the bladder and arteries.

B = False   Elastin is a component of supporting tissue and is absent from epithelia such as the epidermis. Likewise, epithelia do not contain blood vessels, nerves or collagen fibres, which are all components of supporting tissue. Stretch in epithelia is a function of the epithelial cells, a good example being **transitional epithelium**, which allows expansion and contraction of the bladder without losing its impermeability. Elastic recoil of epithelia is dependent on the elastin fibres in the underlying supporting tissue.

C = True   **Tropoelastin** is secreted into the tissues and undergoes polymerisation to form an amorphous mass of elastin. Tropoelastin, unlike tropocollagen, has no cross-banding pattern such as is seen in type I collagen.

D = True   **Fibrillin** is closely associated with elastin in its polymerised form. Fibrillin is a structural **glycoprotein** that forms microfibrils 8–12 nm in diameter. Fibrillin microfibrils are essential for the polymerisation of tropoelastin to form elastin in the tissues and may have a role in binding the tropoelastin molecules together.

E = False   Tropoelastin, like tropocollagen and most of the structural glycoproteins of supporting tissue, is a product of **fibroblasts**. In the resting state these cells have scanty cytoplasm and nuclei that appear inactive. However, during active synthesis, such as during wound healing, the nuclei become enlarged with prominent nucleoli. The cytoplasm is expanded and there is plentiful rough endoplasmic reticulum, as one would expect in a protein-secreting cell.

A = False   This is **transitional epithelium**, which is found only in the renal pelves, ureters, bladder and urethra. Keratinisation is only seen in stratified squamous epithelium. Note, however, that in some pathological conditions, such as chronic inflammation, the bladder may undergo **squamous metaplasia**, where transitional epithelium is replaced by stratified squamous epithelium.

B = True The surface cells, known as **umbrella cells**, are large, often overlapping several cells in the deeper layers. When the bladder fills with urine, the transitional epithelium stretches and the surface cells become flattened. By means of specialised membrane structures, known as **plaques** or **asymmetrical unit membrane**, the umbrella cells can increase their surface area so that they can form a coherent layer on the surface of the epithelium, maintaining the permeability barrier between the urine and the blood in the mucosal capillaries.

C = False Binucleate cells are only found in the surface layer, the umbrella cells, where they are common (none are seen in this micrograph). The umbrella cells are also distinctive because of their large size and scalloped outline. The surface plasma membrane is also thicker than in other cells and stains densely (see B above).

D = False Mucus-secreting cells are not found in transitional epithelium. The epithelium acts as an impermeable barrier between urine and blood and has no secretory function.

E = True Transitional epithelium is normally two to five layers thick. When the bladder is full and the epithelium is stretched it is two to three cells thick and in the relaxed state it is four to five cells thick. Most specimens of bladder seen on histological slides are in the relaxed state. An important feature of malignant tumours of the bladder, **transitional cell carcinomas**, is that the epithelium becomes thicker and is usually more than seven layers thick. However, the thickness of transitional epithelium can also be increased in response to inflammation (**cystitis**), often termed **reactive hyperplasia**.

PAPER 3	ANSWER 3.5

A = False No lymphocytes are normally found in brain tissue although they may infiltrate the brain in inflammatory conditions such as **viral encephalitis**. This cell is one of the support cells (**glial cells**) of the central nervous system tissue. All of the smaller nuclei in this micrograph represent support cells and these cells, with their unstained cytoplasm, are most likely to be **oligodendrocytes**. Oligodendrocytes are often found in close apposition to the nuclei of neurones as well as scattered through the brain tissue.

B = True This cell is a **neurone**, and is recognisable as such because of its large nucleus, prominent nucleolus and plentiful cytoplasm. The cytoplasm of neurones contains plentiful rough endoplasmic reticulum (rER) which is known as **Nissl bodies**. Other staining techniques, such as the Nissl technique, make the Nissl body much more prominent. The axons and dendrites of the neurone cannot be individually identified by this staining method.

C = False   The cell marked **Z** is a glial cell, most probably an **astrocyte**. Astrocytes are cells with multiple cytoplasmic processes but only neurones have **axons** and **dendrites**. Astrocytes provide mechanical support for neurones as well as metabolic support in that they control the exchange of metabolites between the blood and neurones. Astrocytes also contribute to the **blood–brain barrier**.

D = True   The **neuropil** consists of unmyelinated axons, dendrites and the processes of glial cells. The axons are unmyelinated because they are very close to the neurone cell bodies but become myelinated as they enter the white matter of the medulla.

E = False   This is **cerebral cortex** or **grey matter**. The **medulla** or **white matter** contains no neurone cell bodies, consisting of nerve axons, many of which are arranged into **tracts** and most of which are myelinated. Also in the medulla are glial cells and their processes. The myelinated nature of the nerve fibres in the medulla gives the medulla its white appearance.

PAPER 3   ANSWER 3.6

A = True   This thin-walled somewhat irregular vascular channel can be identified as a small **lymphatic**. The lumen is wide compared to the very thin wall in which only very occasional smooth muscle cells are seen. The lumen of this lymphatic contains precipitated **plasma proteins**, which are pale pink (**eosinophilic**) in colour, but in contrast to the other vascular structures in the micrograph there are no erythrocytes in the lumen of the vessel. Some lymphatics, especially close to sites of inflammation, contain lymphocytes in their lumina but in many cases, as here, no lymphocytes are seen.

B = False   This blood vessel is a **venule** and can be identified as such by its wide diameter in relation to the thickness of the wall. The wall consists of one or two layers of smooth muscle cells and the endothelium is barely identifiable. The vessel (**Z**) at the middle left of the micrograph is a small arteriole with a thicker wall consisting of two to three layers of smooth muscle cells enclosing a narrower lumen.

C = False   **Fenestrated endothelium** is found only in the capillaries of certain organs such as the small intestine, kidney and endocrine glands. The fenestrations in the capillary endothelium of these organs facilitates the exchange of materials between blood and the tissue. The endothelium in veins, venules, arteries and arterioles is continuous and almost always flattened. The exception to this rule is the **high endothelial venules** (HEV) of lymphoid tissue where the endothelium is cuboidal. These HEV represent the sites where lymphocytes leave the circulatory system and enter lymphoid tissue.

D = False   This is a small arteriole. The wall consists of two to three layers of
             smooth muscle cells without distinct elastic layers, lined by a thin
             endothelium and surrounded by a barely visible *adventitia*.
             Elastic arteries, in contrast, consist of multiple layers of smooth
             muscle cells sandwiched between concentric *elastic laminae*.
             Elastic arteries include the aorta and its major branches as well
             as the larger pulmonary vessels. The elastic lamina in these
             vessels is important for recoil of the vessels during diastole, thus
             averaging out the blood pressure.

E = False   Most lymphatics of this size or larger contain delicate valves
             consisting of collagenous tissue. These valves prevent the
             backwards flow of lymph in the vessels. Lymph flow is dependent
             on the pumping action caused by movement of adjacent muscles
             as well as gravity. However, the valves of small lymphatic vessels
             are seldom seen in tissue sections in practice, either because
             they are destroyed during tissue preparation or because of an
             unfavourable plane of section.

A = True   The hair shaft is formed of three layers of epithelial cells. The
             inner layer of cells gives rise to the moderately keratinised inner
             part of the hair follicle known as the *medulla*. The thickest layer
             of the hair shaft is the *cortex*, which is highly keratinised. The
             outer layer or *cuticle* of the hair consists of keratin plates that
             overlap each other. The medulla may not be distinguishable in
             fine hairs, as is the case here where only cuticle and cortex are
             seen.

B = False   The hair shaft is produced by the *hair matrix*, a mass of cells
             found at the base of the hair follicle. Along with the *dermal
             papilla*, the hair matrix (not seen in this transverse view) forms
             the *hair bulb*. The dermal papilla is a vascular extension of the
             dermis that forms the centre of the hair bulb. The hair matrix is
             made up of dividing epithelial cells, which become continuous
             with the various layers of the hair shaft and root sheath. The
             internal root sheath is the strongly stained layer internal to the
             external root sheath (see C below) and consists of epithelial
             cells containing plentiful *keratohyaline granules*.

C = False   **X** is a layer of epithelial cells known as the external root sheath.
             The external root sheath takes no part in formation of the hair
             shaft but represents a continuation of the basal layer of the
             surface epithelium (the epidermis). Occasional *melanocytes* may
             be found in this layer but the bulk of the melanocytes which
             produce the melanin which gives hair its colour are found among
             the epithelial cells of the hair matrix.

D = True   This thick specialised basement membrane is known as the
            glassy membrane. It is a continuation, albeit of somewhat
            different structure, of the basement membrane which separates
            the dermis from the epidermis. The glassy membrane separates
            the epithelial cells of the external root sheath from the underlying
            connective tissue sheath that surrounds the follicle.

E = True   Curly hair may be produced by curved or bent follicles and
            straight hair by straight follicles. However, the straightness or
            curliness of the hair is also determined by the cross-sectional
            shape of the hair shaft: individuals of Mongol race have round
            hairs in cross-section whilst those of Caucasians are oval and
            Negroes kidney-bean shaped, giving rise to straight, wavy and
            tightly curled hair respectively.

PAPER 3	ANSWER 3.8

A = True   The surface layer of **synovium** is composed of **synovial cells**
            (**synovocytes**). These cells are of mesenchymal origin. There are
            two types of synovocytes. **Type A synovocytes**, which are most
            numerous, resemble macrophages and contain numerous
            lysosomes and an extensive Golgi apparatus. **Type B
            synovocytes**, which contain plentiful rough endoplasmic
            reticulum, are specialised fibroblasts.

B = False   Synovial cells do not rest on a basement membrane, nor do they
            have the characteristic intercellular connections of epithelial cells.
            Thus synovium does not have the characteristic features of
            epithelia. Cytokeratin, the intermediate filament found in all
            epithelia, is also absent from synovial cells.

C = True   **Synovial fluid**, which cushions and lubricates the articular
            surfaces of joints, is secreted by type B synovocytes. The fluid
            consists of **hyaluronic acid** and glycoproteins that form a viscid
            fluid. The secretory function of type B synovocytes is consistent
            with their extensive rough endoplasmic reticulum, a constant
            feature of cells which secrete substantial amounts of protein.

D = True   Synovial fluid and synovial lining are found in all synovial joints,
            which includes the facet joints of the spinous processes, most of
            the joints of the limbs, the temporomandibular joints and many
            others. Synovial joints are also known as **diarthroses**. Non-
            synovial joints include **syndesmoses** or fibrous joints such as
            those between the skull plates of babies, **synchondroses** or
            primary cartilagenous joints, and **symphyses** or secondary
            cartilagenous joints. The only synchondrosis in humans is the
            joint between the first rib and the sternum. Symphyses are found
            at the pubic symphysis and the intervertebral joints.

E = False   The supporting tissue of the synovium contains plentiful capillaries, which allow diffusion of oxygen, metabolites and carbon dioxide between the blood and the joint fluid and tissues. The supporting tissue may contain more or less collagen or may consist largely of adipose tissue in intra-articular fat pads. Synovium with less, more loosely arranged collagen is known as *areolar synovium*, while *fibrous synovium*, as in this case, has coarse bundles of collagen.

A = False   *Peyer's patches* are groups of *lymphoid follicles* found in the lamina propria of the small bowel. As with organised lymphoid tissue elsewhere, the follicles are composed mainly of B lymphocytes. In this micrograph, **X** marks the *mantle zone* of the follicle, a rim of small resting B cells which surrounds the activated B cells of the *germinal centre*. Peyer's patches form part of the immune defence system of the gastrointestinal tract, known as *GALT* (*gut-associated lymphoid tissue*). GALT in turn is part of *MALT* (*mucosa-associated lymphoid tissue*) which protects mucosal surfaces in the gastrointestinal, respiratory and urogenital tracts.

B = False   In general, lymphocytes found in MALT recirculate to mucosal sites, while lymphocytes from peripheral sites such as the skin migrate back to those sites. For instance, Peyer's patch lymphocytes migrate from Peyer's patches to mesenteric lymph nodes, to spleen and back to mucosal sites, including the gastrointestinal tract mucosa, the lung and the breast in lactating women.

C = False   Peyer's patches are found only in the duodenum, jejunum and ileum and are most prominent in the distal part of the ileum. Similar but smaller lymphoid aggregates are found in the large bowel but these are not called Peyer's patches. In the large bowel these lymphoid aggregates are mainly situated in the submucosa and lower part of the mucosa.

D = True   The Peyer's patch forms a dome-shaped area in the mucosa that is covered by epithelium specialised for antigen uptake. The epithelial cells in these areas are low columnar to cuboidal and few goblet cells are seen. Instead, specialised *M cells* are scattered throughout the epithelium. These are antigen capture cells and have surface microfolds rather than the microvilli found on enterocytes. Many lymphocytes are also seen within the epithelium in these areas, as is well demonstrated in this micrograph.

E = False   Peyer's patches are sites of antigen sampling. Antigen captured by M cells is transported through the epithelium, taken up by macrophages and presented to lymphocytes. B cells responding to this antigen migrate to mesenteric lymph nodes and the spleen where they complete activation and clonal expansion. The activated B cells, *immunoblasts*, recirculate to the lamina propria of the gut where they mature into *plasma cells*. Most of the plasma cells of MALT are committed to IgA production.

A = True   *Kulchitsky cells*, which are part of the *diffuse neuroendocrine system*, are found scattered as single cells and small clusters throughout the epithelium of the respiratory tract in a similar fashion to those found in the gastrointestinal tract. These cells are found resting against the basement membrane between the bases of adjacent epithelial cells where their secretions can easily pass into the underlying capillaries.

B = False   Neuroendocrine cells contain cytoplasmic *dense core granules*. These are membrane-bound vesicles with a rounded electron-dense central area surrounded by a clear zone, hence the term 'dense core'. These granules characteristically contain the protein chromogranin A, and antibodies to chromogranin A can be used to identify neuroendocrine cells using immunoperoxidase techniques. Similarly, antibodies to the hormones within the granules, such as *serotonin*, *bombesin, calcitonin* and *leu-enkephalin*, could be used to highlight these cells. *Synaptic vesicles* are found in nerve cells in the ends of axons and dendrites. In conjunction with the sympathetic nervous system, the neuroendocrine cell products (locally acting hormones) play a role in the regulation of smooth muscle tone in the airways. The tone of the smooth muscle determines the diameter of the airway and therefore the flow of air.

C = True   In the distal bronchioles *Clara cells* are prominent, entirely replacing the mucus-secreting *goblet cells* found in the larger airways. Clara cells act as reserve cells, dividing to replace apoptotic epithelial cells as part of normal cell turnover and repair. Clara cells also secrete a component of *surfactant* and are able to detoxify noxious substances. In the upper airways, goblet cells are easily identified by their clear goblet-shaped collection of mucous in the apical cytoplasm..

D = False   This is the wall of an *alveolus*, one of many seen in this micrograph. The alveolar wall is lined on both sides by flattened epithelial cells known as *type I pneumocytes*. In addition bulbous *type II pneumocytes* are found at the junctions of alveolar walls. Type II pneumocytes contain *lamellar bodies* and are responsible for the secretion of a major component of *surfactant*. Surfactant reduces the surface tension of the alveolar wall and prevents collapse of the alveolus during expiration. Endothelial calls are found within the alveolar walls lining the extensive network of capillaries found there.

E = True   The walls of **bronchioles** consist of an inner lining of epithelium
separated from the smooth muscle layer **Z** by a loose supporting
tissue layer known as the **lamina propria**. The smooth muscle
layer consists of smooth muscle cells arranged in a circular
fashion. The walls of bronchioles contain no cartilage. In the
trachea hyaline cartilage forms C-shaped rings. In the larger
bronchi these C-shaped rings give way to irregular cartilagenous
plates which become smaller in smaller bronchi until they
disappear completely in the bronchioles.

A = True   Although the muscle layer, the **muscularis propria**, of the rest of
the gastrointestinal tract consists entirely of **smooth muscle**, in
the upper one-third of the oesophagus there is a mixture of
smooth and **striated** (**skeletal**) **muscle** (not identifiable in this
low-magnification micrograph). As the initiation of swallowing is a
voluntary action, this arrangement explains itself. The skeletal
muscle component is prominent in the uppermost part of the
oesophagus and is reduced distally until by the middle one-third,
the muscularis propria is composed entirely of smooth muscle
and the movement of food through the rest of the oesophagus is
involuntary.

B = False   The epithelium of the oesophagus in humans is a **stratified
squamous epithelium**, which is not keratinised. In some animal
species with a very coarse diet, the epithelium may be
keratinised. No digestive processes occur in the oesophagus. The
epithelium is thus adapted for the passage of food to the
stomach. The stratified nature of the epithelium, as in the skin,
oropharynx and other areas of the body, is designed to resist
abrasion.

C = False   The outer layer of the oesophageal wall is a layer of loose
supporting tissue called the **adventitia**, which merges with the
surrounding supporting tissue of the posterior mediastinum. That
part of the gastrointestinal tract found within the abdominal cavity
has a surface mesothelial layer (the **visceral peritoneum**) and is
called the **serosa** of the gastrointestinal tract.

D = True   As in the rest of the gastrointestinal tract, clusters of
parasympathetic ganglion cells are found between the two
layers of the muscularis propria. These form the **myenteric** or
Auerbach's plexus, which, together with the **submucosal** or
Meissner's plexus, regulates the motility of the gastrointestinal
tract. The motility and secretions of the gastrointestinal tract are
also influenced by locally produced hormones that are secreted
by the **neuroendocrine cells** scattered throughout the tract.

E = True   **Seromucinous glands** similar in appearance to mixed salivary glands are found in the **submucosa** of the oesophagus, in particular in the upper and lower thirds. These glands empty their secretions onto the epithelial surface via a duct. The secretions serve, along with saliva, to lubricate the passage of food along the oesophagus.

A = True   **X** marks an **islet of Langerhans**, which produces the polypeptide hormones **glucagon**, **insulin**, **somatostatin**, **vasoactive intestinal peptide** (VIP) and **pancreatic polypeptide** (PP). The islets of Langerhans form the endocrine component of the pancreas, a major gland composed of both endocrine and exocrine tissue. The islets of Langerhans are composed of up to 3000 secretory cells arranged in clusters scattered throughout the pancreas. Different cell types in the islets include **alpha cells**, which produce glucagon, **beta cells**, producing insulin, and **delta cells**, which secrete somatostatin.

B = False   **Y** is an **interlobular duct** and carries the products of the exocrine pancreas via the main pancreatic duct to the duodenum. The islets of Langerhans have a very rich capillary network which is in close contact with the endocrine cells and into which the endocrine hormones are secreted. Endocrine glands, also called ductless glands, secrete their products directly into the bloodstream.

C = False   The area marked **Z** is part of the exocrine component of the pancreas made up of **acinar cells**. The acinar cells, in common with other protein-producing cells, are rich in **rough endoplasmic reticulum (rER)**. These cells produce large amounts of digestive enzymes for secretion into the gastrointestinal tract.

D = False   The ductal system of the pancreas consists of small **intercalated ducts** which drain into **intralobular ducts**. These in turn drain into **interlobular ducts** as represented here by **Y**. These are recognisable by their prominent fibrous tissue sheath. Most of the interlobular ducts drain into the **main pancreatic duct** and thence into the duodenum via the **papilla of Vater**. A small proportion of interlobular ducts drain into the duodenum via a small **accessory pancreatic duct**.

E = True   The acinar cells form a roughly spherical **acinus** producing digestive enzymes. These enzymes are synthesised in the plentiful rough endoplasmic reticulum, which is found in the basal part of the cell. The proteins (enzymes) are then transported to the **Golgi apparatus** where final modifications are made to the protein structure and the enzymes are packaged into membrane-

131

bound secretory vesicles. The **zymogen granules** (secretory vesicles) are conveyed to the apical plasma membrane where secretion of their content takes place by **exocytosis**. The enzymes, many of which are secreted in an inactive form to avoid autodigestion, pass from the central lumen of the acinus into the duct system as described above.

A = False   The muscular wall of the upper two-thirds of the ureter consists of two layers of smooth muscle. There is an inner longitudinal layer and an outer circular layer (both actually spirals). In the lower third, this is supplemented by a further outer longitudinal layer. In practice it is difficult to identify the separate layers. No skeletal muscle is found in the ureter.

B = True   **Transitional epithelium** or **urothelium** lines the renal pelves, ureters, urinary bladder, and part of the urethra. It is characterised by its ability to stretch and its impermeability. These features are attributable to the multiplicity of tight junctions between cells, the **umbrella cells**, on the surface and the stratified nature of the epithelium.

C = False   The layer marked **Z** is the **lamina propria**. It carries small blood vessels that supply the epithelium and inner muscle. The major blood supply of the ureter comes from the larger vessels seen in the adventitia (see E below).

D = False   The muscle layer of the ureter is surrounded by a loose **adventitia** made up of supporting tissues (adipose tissue and collagenous tissue). This layer blends in with the surrounding retroperitoneal tissues and is not demarcated by any definite structure. The entire urinary tract is a retroperitoneal structure. The major vessels and nerves run in the adventitia.

E = True   The smooth muscle of the wall of the ureter contracts spontaneously in an ordered fashion to move the urine down the ureter to the bladder. This is similar to the spontaneous contraction or **peristalsis** seen in the smooth muscle of the wall of the gastrointestinal tract and is also known as peristalsis or **vermiculation**.

A = False   The eosinophilic (pink) material in the centre of the follicles is **thyroglobulin** (thyroid **colloid**), a glycoprotein which acts as a storage site for thyroid hormones. Both **T3** and **T4** are stored in the colloid. **Calcitonin** is synthesised and secreted into the blood directly. The **C cells**, which produce calcitonin, are part of the diffuse neuroendocrine system. The calcitonin is found in the C-cell cytoplasm in **dense core granules** prior to secretion. The dense core granules are easily recognised in electron micrographs.

B = False   The activity of the thyroid gland or indeed different parts of the gland may vary according to metabolic needs and the availability of iodine. The thyroid epithelial cells form a simple epithelium and vary from low cuboidal to high columnar according to these variables. Tall columnar epithelium is seen in very active tissue and this effect is exaggerated in **Graves' disease**, an autoimmune condition characterised by marked oversecretion of thyroid hormones giving rise to the clinical condition of **hyperthyroidism**. Similarly, the amount of colloid in the follicles varies and in very active glands (and especially in Graves' disease) the colloid is pale and often has a scalloped outline.

C = True   The **thyroid follicle** is the basic structural unit of the thyroid gland. It consists of a single layer of cuboidal to columnar cells, which trap iodine and synthesise thyroid hormones. The hormones are then stored in the colloid until required. Thyroid hormone secretion is regulated by **thyroid stimulating hormone** (**TSH**) secreted by the anterior pituitary gland.

D = True   The thyroid contains a very extensive network of capillary vessels which course between the follicles. The capillaries have a fenestrated endothelium which presumably facilitates release of T3 and T4 and calcitonin into the circulation.

E = False   **C cells** (**clear cells** or **parafollicular cells**) are difficult if not impossible to identify in normal human thyroid in H & E sections. In other species identification may be easier as clearing of the cytoplasm is more obvious. The C cells are found within the basement membrane of the follicles tucked between the thyroid epithelial cells. The C cells do not extend through the full thickness of the epithelium and are therefore not in contact with the colloid. Also many sections of thyroid tissue will be devoid of C cells as these are only found in the mid-zones of the lateral lobes of the thyroid in humans.

PAPER 3	ANSWER 3.15

A = False   The structure marked **X** is one of two **corpora amylacea** seen in this micrograph. These lamellated structures formed of glycoproteins are seen in increasing numbers with age and are rarely found in young boys.

B = False   The glandular epithelium consists of two cell layers. The luminal layer is made up of tall cuboidal or columnar cells. The basal layer, which is often incomplete, consists of flattened epithelial cells, which may serve as stem or reserve cells.

133

C = False Lipofuscin granules are characteristically seen in the epithelium of the **seminal vesicle** and provide a useful means of differentiating between prostate and seminal vesicle tissue in small core biopsies of the prostate, a method increasingly used to diagnose **prostatic adenocarcinoma**.

D = True The **fibrinolysin** and other hydrolytic enzymes found in the prostatic secretions liquefy the coagulated semen in the vagina.

E = True The **stroma** of the prostate contains plentiful smooth muscle fibres as well as collagenous supporting tissue. These smooth muscle cells contract during ejaculation to propel the contents of the gland into the penile urethra.

PAPER 3   ANSWER 3.16

A = False This is **early proliferative phase** endometrium. In the early proliferative phase of the menstrual cycle, the glands begin as quite short and sparse but become longer and straight during this part of the cycle owing to proliferation (cell division by **mitosis**) of both glandular epithelial cells and **stromal cells**. As this proliferation continues the glands become coiled during the later part of the proliferative phase. When proliferation ceases at the time of ovulation the glands still have a coiled appearance but the epithelial cells show features of secretion. **Secretory phase endometrium** is characterised by coiled glands, secretory material within the cytoplasm of the epithelial cells and/or the lumina of the glands, absence of mitoses and changes in the stroma and blood vessels.

B = False This is a **mitotic figure (metaphase)**, which characterises the proliferative phase of the cycle. **Subnuclear vacuoles** appear in the early days of the secretory phase, when the epithelial cells begin to produce the secretions, consisting mainly of glycogen, ready to nourish the early embryo should fertilisation and implantation take place. These secretory vacuoles move up to a supranuclear position and are then released into the gland lumen in the late secretory phase.

C = False The cells indicated by **Y** are the **endometrial stromal cells**. The stroma of the endometrium is also hormone responsive and proliferates along with the glands to form a thick layer during the proliferative phase. A stromal mitotic figure can be seen in the mid left area of the micrograph. Endometrial stromal cells are derived from mesoderm. The cells have ovoid nuclei and indistinct, scanty cytoplasm. The myometrium, the thick smooth muscle layer of the uterus, lies deep to the endometrium and is not seen in this micrograph.

D = True   The epithelium is a pseudostratified columnar epithelium with cilia, making up tubular glands which are straight during the early proliferative phase but become coiled in the later part of the proliferative phase.

E = False   The only way to tell from the endometrium that ovulation has occurred is when **subnuclear (basal) vacuoles** appear. These are clear areas in the lower cytoplasm of the epithelial cells. Subnuclear vacuoles appear within 2 days of ovulation. Proliferation ceases at this stage although an occasional cell can be seen on day 16–17 completing mitosis. At the start of the secretory phase, which begins at the time of ovulation, the glands are already long and coiled.

PAPER 3   ANSWER 3.17

A = False   The epithelium of the **ectocervix X** is a non-keratinising **stratified squamous epithelium**, similar to that found in the vagina and the oesophagus. The epithelial cells often appear to have clear cytoplasm because of their high content of glycogen. This should not be confused with the **koilocytes** seen in **human papillomavirus infection (HPV)** of the ectocervix. Koilocytes also have clear cytoplasm but have very abnormal nuclei and are generally accompanied by other features of HPV infection.

B = False   The **stroma** of the cervix **Y** consists mainly of collagenous supporting tissue as well as blood vessels, nerves and a small amount of smooth muscle. A small number of lymphocytes are also generally seen in the cervical stroma and these are greatly increased and accompanied by other inflammatory cells in **cervicitis** where the cervix is inflamed.

C = True   The **endocervix** is lined by a **simple columnar mucus-secreting epithelium (Z)** which produces the normal **cervical mucus**.

D = False   The epithelium of the **endocervical glands** is the same as the endocervical surface epithelium. These are not true glands but rather folds or clefts of surface epithelium dipping down into the stroma. This micrograph shows the **squamocolumnar junction**, the area where the ectocervix meets the endocervix. Those students who are still awake at this stage will have noticed that an endocervical gland is seen on the right side of the micrograph deep to squamous epithelium. The squamous epithelium has replaced surface endocervical epithelium, a process known as **squamous metaplasia**. Although strictly speaking this is a pathological process, it is in reality so common that it is considered a variant of normal. For this reason this area is often called the **transformation zone**.

E = True   The **Pap smear** is a technique whereby cervical surface epithelium is removed by scraping or brushing the cervix. The

135

material produced is smeared onto a slide and stained by the Papanicolaou method, which allows examination of both ectocervical and endocervical epithelium for premalignant changes. Newer methods of preparation include the '*Thin Prep*' technique, which spreads the epithelial cells in a more even layer on the slide, and various computer software programs which analyse the material for abnormal cells. The transformation zone is the usual place to find precancerous changes

A = True   **X** marks the *amnion*, which is composed of three layers. The *epithelium* is easily recognised and is lying on a thick *basement membrane*, the middle layer. The outer layer of the amnion is the avascular *mesenchymal layer*. This layer, which is slightly disrupted in this micrograph, is derived from *extraembryonic mesoderm*. In this micrograph the mesenchymal layer is not sharply demarcated from the underlying *chorion*.

B = True   The *chorion* component of the membranes is also composed of three layers. The innermost layer, which is adjacent to the mesenchymal layer of the amnion, is the vascular collagenous inner layer. In this micrograph the innermost layer of the chorion and the outermost layer of the amnion are not sharply demarcated and there is no intermediate layer, which is thin in some membranes. The middle layer of the chorion is derived from *trophoblast* and is known as the *trophoblast layer*. The outermost or maternal layer of the chorion is the *decidua capsularis*.

C = True   As mentioned above, the trophoblast layer is the central layer of the chorion.

D = False   The amnion (**X**) consists entirely of fetal tissue. The only maternally derived layer of the entire membranes is the outermost layer of the chorion, the decidua capsularis. All the other layers are of fetal origin.

E = True   The amnion forms the fetal side of the membranes, with the chorion on the maternal side. This is probably obvious from the fact that the outermost layer of a chorion is composed of flattened decidua, the decidua capsularis, which is modified endometrium.

A = True   This structure is the *ciliary body*, part of the uveal tract, the other components being the *iris* anteriorly and the *choroid* posteriorly. The ciliary body is a ring of smooth muscle that bulges into the eye at the junction between the anterior one-sixth and posterior five-sixths of the eye. The ciliary body is composed mainly of smooth muscle, which by contracting and relaxing alters the shape of the **lens**, thus focusing incoming light on the **retina**. The lens is joined to the ciliary body by the **suspensory ligament**, which is often destroyed during histological preparation, as is the case here.

B = False   The epithelium lining the ciliary body consists of a double layer of epithelium, the deeper layer of which is pigmented. This epithelium is continuous with the retina, with the pigmented layer corresponding to the pigmented layer of the retina. However, **photoreceptor cells** (the **rods** and **cones**) are not found in the forward part of the inner layer of the eye. The photosensitive retina terminates at the **ora serrata**.

C = True   The iris represents the anterior part of the uveal tract and is the part of the eye that is most noticeable to the outside observer. The iris lies anterior to the lens and separates the **anterior compartment** of the eye into **anterior** and **posterior chambers**. The iris contains delicate smooth muscle fibres, contraction of which regulates the diameter of the central aperture of the iris in response to the intensity of the incoming light.

D = True   This is the **canal of Schlemm**, which lies in the choroid layer at the outer angle of the anterior chamber. Aqueous humor produced continuously by the ciliary body circulates through the aperture of the iris into the anterior chamber where it drains via the canal of Schlemm into the general circulation. The aqueous humor, by means of this balanced production and reabsorption, is maintained at a pressure of about 15 mmHg. Any upset in this balance causing an increase in the pressure of aqueous fluid, gives rise to the clinical condition of **glaucoma**, an important cause of blindness.

E = True   The anterior compartment of the eye is bounded anteriorly by the **cornea** and posteriorly by the lens and suspensory ligament. The iris divides this anterior compartment into the anterior and posterior chambers, which are filled with **aqueous humor**. The posterior compartment of the eye contains the **vitreous body**.

PAPER 3	ANSWER 3.20

A = False   These are **smooth** or **visceral muscle fibres**. Like skeletal and cardiac muscle fibres they contain both **thin** and **thick contractile filaments (actin** and **myosin** respectively). It is the sliding of thin and thick filaments with respect to each other that causes contraction and relaxation of muscle. In smooth muscle the contractile filaments are arranged in a random orientation in the cell, while in cardiac and skeletal muscle the filaments are arranged in parallel arrays.

B = True These muscle fibres show the pattern of **cross-striations** characteristic of skeletal muscle fibres. The cross-striations are the result of the highly ordered arrangement of the contractile filaments in parallel bundles to form **sarcomeres**. In this micrograph the **I bands** and the **A bands** can easily be seen and the **Z line** is only just visible. Cardiac muscle also has cross-striations but is only found in the heart. Cardiac muscle fibres, unlike skeletal muscle fibres, are branched.

C = True The contractile filaments of smooth muscle are fixed to **focal densities** in the cytoplasm and to **anchoring densities** on the cell membrane. The focal densities are also anchored to the **desmin** intermediate filaments of the **cytoskeleton** of the cell. Thus contraction of the contractile filament is transmitted throughout the cell, which becomes smaller.

D = True The contractile filaments of skeletal muscle are arranged in sarcomeres. A sarcomere is the contractile unit of the myofibrils of skeletal muscle. The sarcomere is defined by a Z line at either end. Adjacent to the Z line is the paler I band consisting of actin filaments only. In the central area of the sarcomere is the darker A band which consists of myosin filaments and varying lengths of actin filaments depending on the state of contraction of the muscle. The **M line** is placed centrally in the A band.

E = False The upper oesophagus is the only part of the gastrointestinal tract where smooth and skeletal muscle are intermingled in this fashion. This is because initiation of swallowing is a voluntary action, while the rest of swallowing is involuntary. Opening and closing of the ileocaecal valve obviously has no voluntary component.

PAPER 3	ANSWER 3.21

A = True The muscle fibres are joined at their blunt ends by a specialised junction known as an **intercalated disc**. The intercalated disc consists of the plasma membranes of adjacent muscle cells folded together in a convoluted pattern and held together by specialised structures (see below). The convoluted membrane structure of the intercalated disc is easy to appreciate in this electron micrograph.

B = True **X** marks a **fascia adherens**. This is one of the specialised connecting structures found in the intercalated disc. The fascia adherens is similar in structure to a **zonula adherens** found in epithelial cells. Actin filaments at the ends of the sarcomeres are attached to the fascia adherens, anchoring adjacent cells to each other and also transmitting the force of contraction between cells. The two other types of connecting structures found at intercalated discs are **desmosomes** and **nexus (gap) junctions** (see below).

C = False   The structure marked **Y** is part of the **_T tubule system_**. In cardiac muscles, the T tubules and sarcoplasmic reticulum form **_triads_** as in skeletal muscle. However, the triads are less regular and well defined than those seen in skeletal muscle and at this power it is not easy to identify the sarcoplasmic reticulum. This T tubule lies immediately adjacent to a **_mitochondrion_**, easily recognised by its inner membrane folded into **_cristae_**. Note also the **_matrix granules_** within the mitochondria. There are multiple mitochondria in this micrograph.

D = True   As in skeletal muscle, **_glycogen granules_** act as a readily available source of energy. Note the large numbers of glycogen granules (small dark dots at this magnification) found in the vicinity of the mitochondria. The glucose which makes up the glycogen is oxidised by oxidative phosphorylation to produce ATP, which is the energy source for muscle contraction.

E = False   Cardiac muscle cells act as a syncytium so that they may contract at the same time in systole. Nexus or gap junctions found at the intercalated discs act as low-resistance conductance channels, allowing cardiac muscle fibres to contract synchronously. Contraction of cardiac muscle fibres is regulated by a specialised conducting system consisting of modified cardiac muscle fibres. At the beginning of systole, a wave of excitation originates at the **_sinoatrial node_** in the right atrium. This wave of excitation passes through the muscle of the atrium to the **_atrioventricular node_**, which then passes the stimulus on to the muscle cells of the ventricles, via the **_atrioventricular bundle_** (**_bundle of His_**). The bundle of His divides into many small branches known as **_Purkinje fibres_**. These ramify through the myocardium permitting simultaneous contraction of the ventricles.

PAPER 3   ANSWER 3.22

A = False   The structure marked **X** and all the neighbouring similar structures are **_microvilli_**. These are found in very large numbers on the luminal surface of the epithelial cells of the small bowel. At the magnifications attainable by light microscopy, the individual microvilli cannot be identified and the microvilli appear as a fuzzy border known as the **_striated border_** along the surface of the epithelium. In contrast, **_cilia_** are longer than microvilli and can be seen by light microscopy as individual structures.

B = True   Microvilli have a central core of **_actin filaments_**. The actin filaments run in parallel along the length of the microvilli and are anchored to the plasma membrane at the tip and to the terminal web at the base of the microvillus (see C below).

C = True   **Y** marks the **terminal web**. This is a specialisation of the **actin cytoskeleton** of the cell. The actin filaments within the microvilli are anchored to it and this in turn is anchored to the **zonula adherens** at the plasma membrane. The zonula adherens is one of the three components of the **junctional complex** binding adjacent epithelial cells to each other. The terminal web is also connected to the cytoskeleton of the cell.

D = True   The microvilli of the small intestine are characteristically covered by a thick layer of glycoproteins known as the **glycocalyx**. The glycocalyx has two functions. One is to protect the epithelial cells from autodigestion. The other function is to trap pancreatic enzymes at the membrane, facilitating enzymatic breakdown of food within the lumen of the bowel.

E = False   Microvilli are found on many cells but are most prominent in the small bowel and in the **proximal convoluted tubule** of the kidney. The bronchi, characteristically, have large numbers of cilia. Cilia have a central core of **microtubules**, which allows them to beat in a coordinated fashion. In the bronchi they move mucus containing entrapped particles up the bronchial tree towards the nasopharynx. Cilia are also found in large numbers on the epithelium of the Fallopian tube. In the Fallopian tube they move the ovum along the tube towards the uterus.

A = False   **X** marks a **type II pneumocyte**. These large rounded cells are easily recognisable by their **lamellar bodies** scattered throughout the cytoplasm. Type I pneumocytes, which line most of the alveolar wall, are flattened cells with extensive thin cytoplasm.

B = True   **Y** is a **lamellar body**. These are membrane-bound structures containing multiple lamellae composed mainly of phospholipids. The major phospholipid within lamellar bodies is **palmitoyl phosphatidylcholine**, one of the components of surfactant. Hence, type II pneumocytes are also known as **surfactant cells**. Type II pneumocytes are usually found at the angle between two alveolae, although this feature is not obvious in the plane of section of this micrograph.

C = False   Type II pneumocytes, as mentioned above, are usually found where two alveolae meet. They bulge into the alveolus, unlike type I pneumocytes, which are flattened and line the majority of the alveolar wall. Type II pneumocytes are not found within the walls of bronchioles, but only in the alveoli.

D = True   **Z** marks a capillary, the lumen of which would be filled with blood in vitro. The capillary is lined by a flattened layer of endothelium.

The endothelial cell nucleus is not visible in this micrograph but the cytoplasm can easily be seen. The endothelium is separated from the type I pneumocyte by a basement membrane, which is also easily identifiable in this micrograph.

E = True As mentioned above, type I pneumocytes have flattened cytoplasm, forming a layer over the alveolar side of the alveolar wall. Where a type I pneumocyte comes into contact with a type II pneumocyte, as seen here, the cytoplasm of the type I pneumocyte extends partly over the surface of the type II pneumocyte. Where the type II pneumocyte is not covered by type I pneumocyte cytoplasm, small stubby microvilli can be identified.

A = True **X** marks the ***mesangium***, which is composed of ***mesangial matrix*** and ***mesangial cells***. The mesangial matrix is similar in composition to basement membrane. The mesangium forms a branched core for the glomerulus, supporting the delicate capillary loops. The edge of the mesangium that faces the capillary loops is lined only by fenestrated endothelium, without an intervening basement membrane. The mesangium is therefore in close contact with the blood flowing through the glomerular capillary loops.

B = False **Y** marks the ***pedicels*** (***podocyte foot processes***) which line the outer side of the glomerular basement membrane. The interdigitating foot processes are separated by a small space that is bridged by a delicate diaphragm (not seen at this magnification). Together with the endothelium and the basement membrane, the pedicels make up part of the glomerular filter. ***Fenestrated endothelium*** lines the capillary side of the glomerular basement membrane as can easily be seen in this micrograph. The fenestrations in the capillary endothelium are rather larger than at other sites of the body, facilitating the filtration mechanism of the glomerulus.

C = True The structure marked **Z** is the capillary basement membrane. It consists of three layers. The central electron-dense layer is the ***lamina densa***, which is the most obvious part of the basement membrane. On either side of the lamina densa are narrow lucid layers known as the ***lamina lucida interna*** (facing the endothelium) and the ***lamina lucida externa*** (facing the podocyte foot processes). It is thought that the basement membrane of the glomerulus is elaborated by both endothelial cells and podocytes. It is much thicker than most other basement membranes in the body.

D = False   The area marked **W** is ***Bowman's space***, which is filled with the plasma ultrafiltrate in vitro. Blood is found within the capillary loops of the glomerulus, that is to say on the side of the glomerular basement membrane lined by fenestrated endothelium. The plasma ultrafiltrate in Bowman's space flows into the ***proximal convoluted tubule*** and through the tubular system, where it is converted into urine by selective exchange of ions and water. In the tubules, small molecules such as glucose and amino acids are also reabsorbed. Other substances such as hydrogen and potassium ions are secreted into the tubules.

E = True   The mesangium contains mesangial cells. These cells, which may be derived from ***pericytes***, have various functions including phagocytosis. In certain types of ***glomerulonephritis***, mesangial cells appear to phagocytose immune complexes deposited within the glomerulus. Mesangial cells contain cytoplasmic ***actin*** and ***myosin filaments***, which gives them the capability to contract, thus modifying the diameter of the glomerular capillaries. They also secrete vasoactive substances, which further modify the diameter of the capillary lumina. These two latter functions of mesangial cells can control the capillary blood flow.

PAPER 4

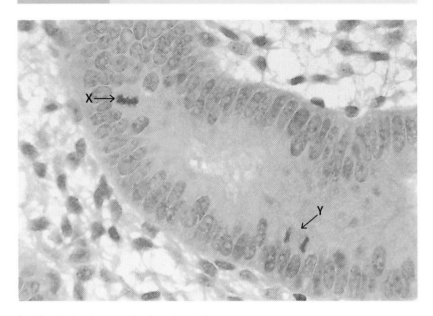

In this photomicrograph of endometrium:

A   The cell marked **X** is in the anaphase stage of mitotic division.

B   The cell marked **Y** is in the second meiotic division.

C   The chromatids in the cell marked **X** have not yet separated from each other.

D   DNA reduplication occurs in the phase immediately after the phase shown in the cell marked **Y**.

E   The mitotic spindle is dismantled immediately after the phase shown in **X**.

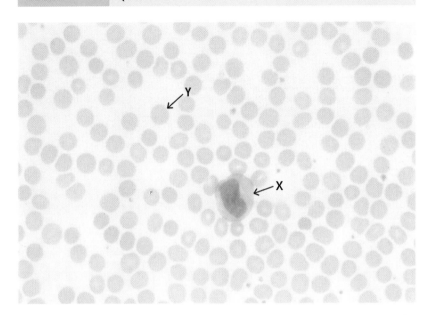

In this micrograph of a peripheral blood smear:

A   The cell marked **X** is a basophil.

B   The cell marked **X** has cytoplasmic granules.

C   The cell marked **Y** has a lifespan of approximately 120 days.

D   The cell marked **X** is related to the Kupffer cells of the liver.

E   The cell marked **Y** contains the protein spectrin.

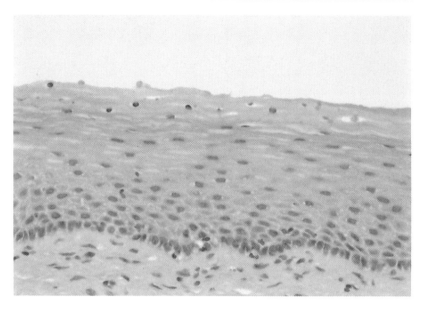

The epithelium shown in this high-power photomicrograph:

A   Is of the type that lines the uterine cervix.

B   Would have dividing cells (mitotic figures) in all layers.

C   Has great tensile strength due to the many desmosomes joining adjacent cells.

D   Is transitional epithelium.

E   Contains desmin intermediate filaments.

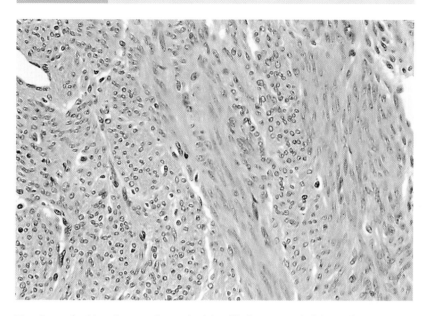

The tissue in this micrograph can be identified as smooth (visceral) muscle because:

A   The muscle cells are arranged in fasciculi.

B   Cross-striations are seen in the cytoplasm.

C   Many branched fibres are seen.

D   The nuclei are centrally orientated in the cells.

E   Both elongated and rounded nuclei are seen.

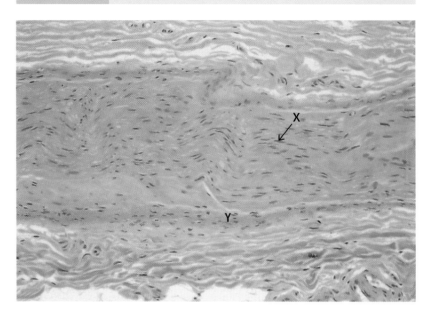

In this medium-power photomicrograph of peripheral nerve:

A The structure marked **X** is a nerve cell nucleus.

B **Y** indicates the perineurium.

C This nerve can easily be identified as an autonomic nerve.

D This is a non-myelinated nerve fibre.

E This nerve consists only of afferent nerve fibres.

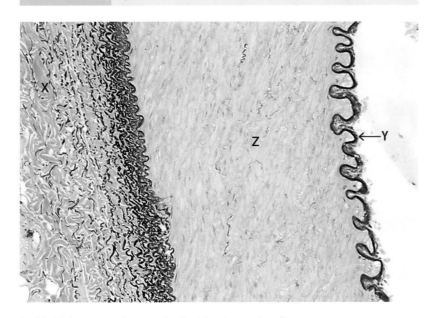

In this high-power micrograph of a blood vessel wall:

A   The structure marked **X** is composed mainly of smooth muscle cells.

B   The structure marked **Y** is the internal elastic lamina.

C   This is the wall of an elastic artery.

D   The tunica media is marked by **Z**.

E   The tunica intima consists mainly of elastic tissue.

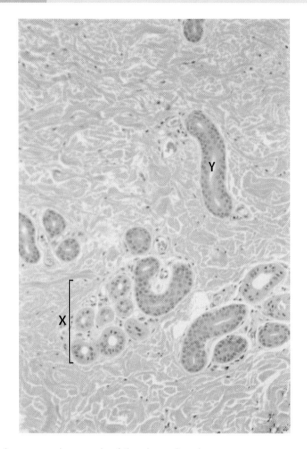

In this high-power micrograph of the deep dermis:

A   The structure marked **X** is usually associated with a hair follicle.

B   The structure marked **X** is found mainly in axillary and genital skin.

C   The structure marked **X** secretes a watery fluid.

D   The structure marked **Y** opens onto the skin surface.

E   Secretion takes place in this structure by decapitation of the secretory cells.

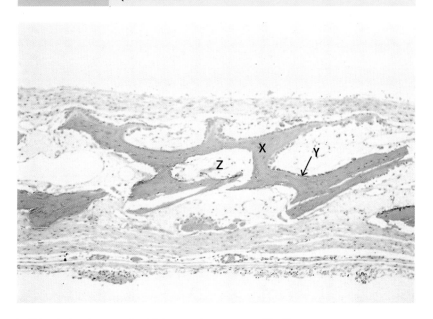

In this photomicrograph of intramembranous ossification:

A   **X** marks a centre of ossification.

B   The cells marked **Y** lay down osteoid which becomes progressively mineralised.

C   Bone formation of this type would typically be seen in the femur of a developing fetus.

D   The area marked **Z** will become colonised by haemopoietic cells.

E   The bones thus formed enlarge during childhood at the epiphyseal growth plate.

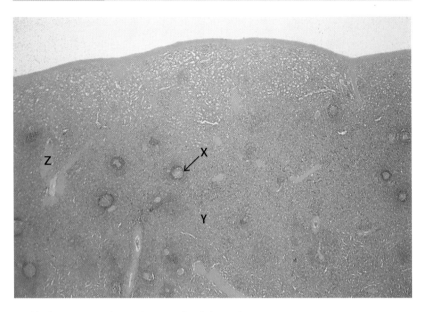

In this low-power photomicrograph of the spleen:

A   The structure marked **X** consists of lymphocytes.

B   The area marked **Y** contains sheathed capillaries.

C   The cords of Bilroth are found in the area marked **X**.

D   The area marked **X** has a marginal zone.

E   The structure marked **Z** divides the spleen into well-defined lobes.

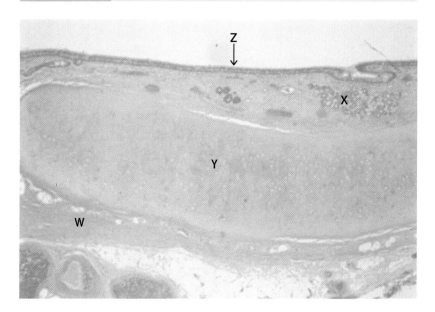

In this micrograph of trachea:

A   The structure marked **X** is part of the thyroid gland.

B   The structure marked **Y** consists of fibrocartilage.

C   The lining epithelium marked **Z** is a stratified squamous epithelium.

D   The trachealis muscle lies in the area marked **W**.

E   The epithelium rests on a thick basement membrane.

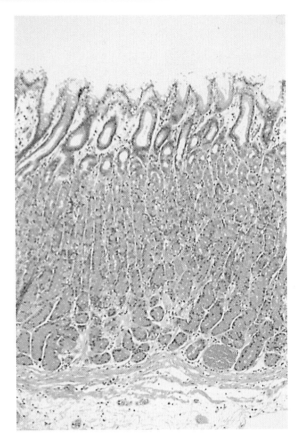

This photomicrograph of gastric mucosa is recognisable as body of the stomach rather than the pyloric antrum because:

A   The mid-portion of the glands contain plentiful parietal cells.

B   The surface epithelium consists of mucus-secreting cells.

C   The bases of the glands are lined by Paneth cells.

D   The glands are straight tubular glands.

E   Most of the cells at the bases of the glands are of the neuroendocrine type.

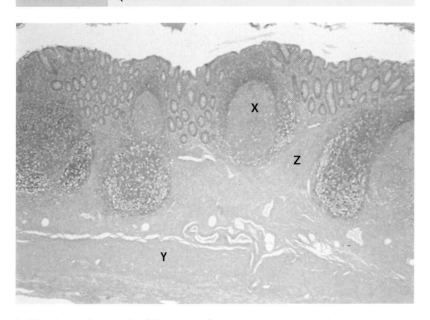

In this photomicrograph of the appendix:

A   The mucosa has a similar structure to the ileum.

B   The structure marked **X** is generally more prominent in elderly than in young individuals.

C   The structure marked **Y** consists of three distinct layers of smooth muscle.

D   Seromucinous glands are found in the area marked **Z**.

E   Parietal cells are scattered throughout the epithelium.

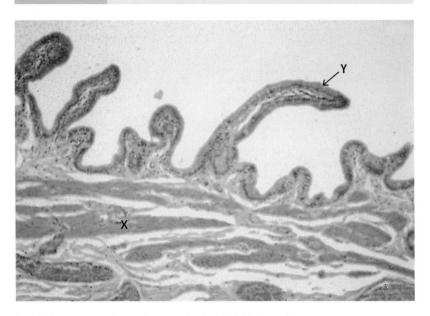

In this low-power photomicrograph of gall bladder wall:

A   The muscle coat of the gall bladder (marked **X)** is arranged in two distinct layers.

B   The lining epithelium **Y** consists of a stratified columnar epithelium.

C   The mucosa is flat when distended.

D   The epithelium of the gall bladder secretes bile into the lumen.

E   The gall bladder contracts in response to the hormone glucagon.

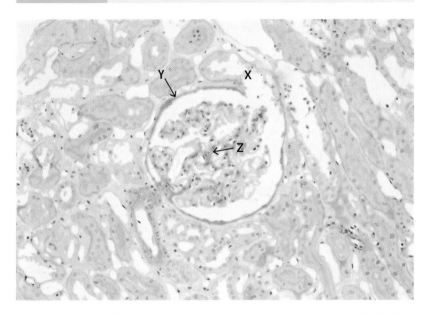

In this high-power photomicrograph of a renal corpuscle stained by the PAS stain:

A   The area marked **X** is the urinary pole of the corpuscle.

B   The structure marked **Y** is Bowman's capsule.

C   The cells lining the structure marked **Y** are known as podocytes.

D   The area marked **Z** consists of mesangial cells and matrix.

E   The glomerular capillary loops are lined by fenestrated endothelium.

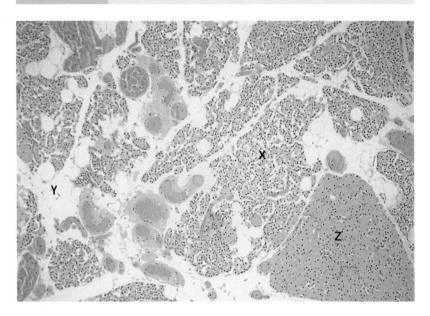

In this micrograph of parathyroid gland:

A The cells marked **X** synthesise and secrete parathormone.

B A normal adult parathyroid gland includes less than 5% of the tissue marked **Y**.

C The epithelial tissue of a normal adult parathyroid gland consists almost entirely of cells of the type marked **X**.

D An electron micrograph of the cells marked **Z** would show numerous mitochondria in the cytoplasm.

E A normal adult may have up to six parathyroid glands.

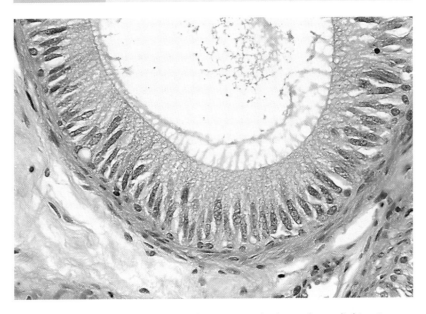

This high-power photomicrograph of a structure in the male genital tract can be identified as:

A   A seminiferous tubule because spermatogonia are clearly identifiable.

B   Part of the epididymis because the stereocilia can be identified.

C   Part of the prostatic urethra because it is lined by pseudostratified columnar epithelium.

D   Part of the rete testis because it is lined by tall columnar epithelium.

E   Part of a seminiferous tubule because Leydig cells can be seen surrounding the tubule.

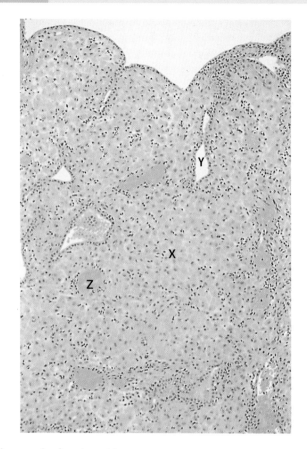

In this micrograph of endometrium:

A   The cells in the area marked **X** are syncytiotrophoblast cells.

B   The structure marked **Y** is a chorionic villus.

C   The endometrial stromal cells are the main source of progestagens in early pregnancy.

D   Decidualisation of the endometrium is seen only in pregnancy.

E   The structure marked **Z** is a spiral artery.

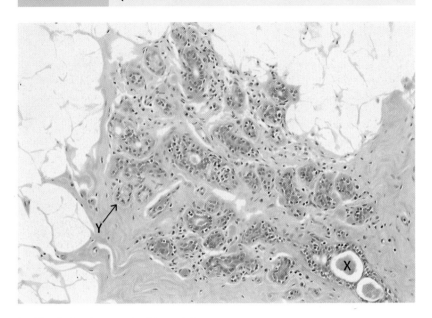

In this photomicrograph of breast tissue:

A   The structure marked **X** is a lactiferous duct.

B   The structure shown here is a terminal duct–lobular unit.

C   The epithelium lining **Y** is made up of two cell layers.

D   Some of the epithelial cells lining the ducts contain actin.

E   During pregnancy, the breast acini enlarge greatly in preparation for lactation.

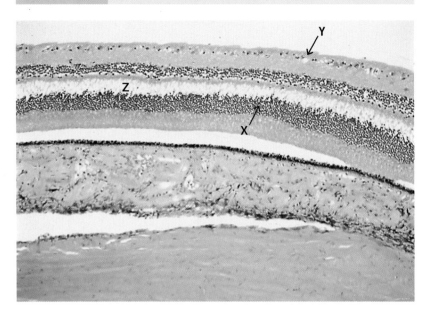

In this photomicrograph of the posterior wall of the eye:

A The cell bodies of the rods and cones are found in the layer marked **X**.

B The layer marked **Y** is separated from the vitreous body by a layer of epithelial cells.

C Small blood vessels run in the layer marked **Z**.

D Müller cells are found in the layers marked **X** and **Y**.

E Nerve fibres run in the layer marked **Y**.

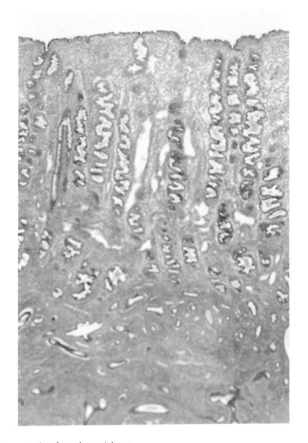

In this micrograph of endometrium:

A   The saw-tooth outline of the glands is typical of early proliferative endometrium.

B   The endometrial stroma consists of smooth muscle cells.

C   The endometrial stroma contains spiral arterioles.

D   Secretions within the lumen of the glands are common in the follicular phase of the menstrual cycle.

E   The lower part of the endometrium produces secretions throughout the menstrual cycle.

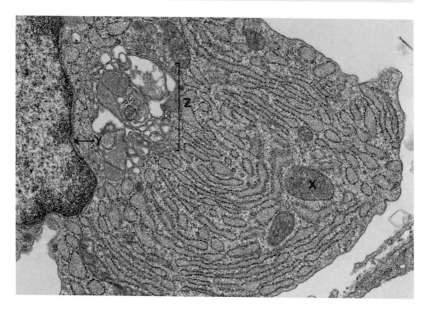

In this medium-power electron micrograph of a cell:

A   The structure marked **X** is a mitochondrion.

B   The cytoplasm is packed with rough endoplasmic reticulum.

C   The structure marked **Y** is a double lipid bilayer membrane.

D   The structure marked **Y** is interrupted by pores.

E   The structure marked **Z** is the site of energy production.

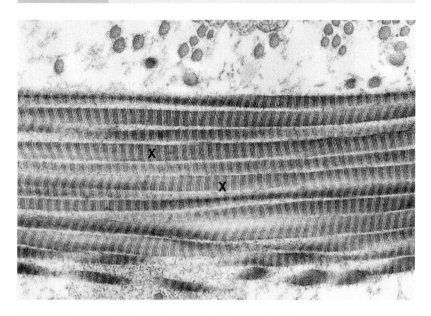

In this high-power electron micrograph of supporting tissue:

A   The structures marked **X** are composed of type IV collagen.

B   The structures marked **X** are made up of tropocollagen molecules.

C   The cross-banding pattern has a periodicity of 64 nm.

D   The structures marked **X** are synthesised by macrophages.

E   The structures marked **X** are prominent in hyaline cartilage.

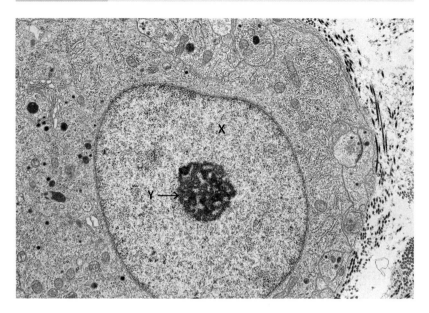

In this medium-power electron micrograph of part of a ganglion cell:

A   The area marked **X** is composed of heterochromatin.

B   The structure marked **X** is surrounded by a double bilayered lipid membrane.

C   The structure marked **Y** is the site of ribosomal RNA synthesis.

D   Histone proteins are not found in the area marked **X**.

E   Ribosome protein synthesis takes place in the area marked **Y**.

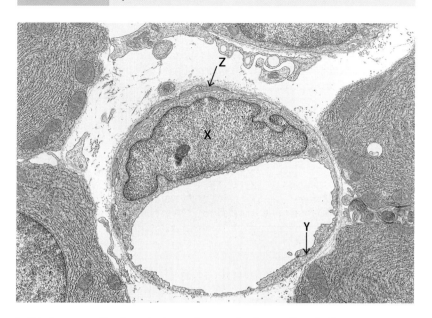

In this low-magnification electron micrograph of a capillary in the pancreas:

A   The structure marked **X** is the nucleus of an endothelial cell.

B   The structure marked **Y** is an intercellular junction.

C   The structure marked **Z** is a smooth muscle cell.

D   The endothelial cells are metabolically inert.

E   The endothelial cells contain Birbeck granules.

A = False   This cell is in **metaphase**, the second stage of mitotic division. At this stage the paired **chromatids** are lined up at the equator of the cell (also known as the **metaphase plate**) prior to separation. The **microtubules** of the **cell spindle** anchor the paired chromatids in place at this stage, prior to drawing one member of each pair to the opposite poles of the cells.

B = False   This is **anaphase**, the third phase of mitosis. Although the second meitoic division may have a similar stage with a similar appearance, this cannot be meiosis. Meiotic division only occurs in the germ cells: the **oocytes** in the ovary in females and the **spermatocytes** of the testis of the male. Meiosis results in the production of **haploid** germ cells, each containing half of the usual number of chromosomes (23 in humans). Two haploid germ cells (one ovum and one spermatozoon) fuse to form a **diploid** zygote, which has the usual complement of chromosomes (46, or 23 pairs, in humans). Cell division in all other cells of the body must be by mitosis. Mitotic cell division produces two diploid daughter cells.

C = True   In metaphase the reduplicated chromosomes (the chromatids) are joined to each other at the **centromere**. Separation of the chromatids occurs in **anaphase**, the third stage of mitosis, when one of each pair is drawn to the opposite poles of the cell.

D = False   Reduplication of the DNA occurs in **S phase** of the cell cycle. In S (or synthesis) phase each chromosome is copied. The cell then passes into G_2 **phase**, which is usually quite short. The four stages of **M phase** then follow (**prophase**, **metaphase**, **anaphase**, **telophase** in that order). The daughter cells of the mitotic division then spend a period of time in G_1 **phase** before DNA synthesis starts again. The time in G_1 phase depends on the type of cell and the circumstances. For example, epithelial cells in normal skin would be expected to have a long G_1 phase but a much shorter G_1 phase during wound healing.

E = False   The mitotic spindle is dismantled at the end of telophase, the fourth stage of mitosis. The mitotic spindle is made up of **chromosome** (or **kinetochore**) **microtubules** and **interpolar microtubules** attached to the paired **centrioles** at opposite poles of the cell. The chromosome microtubules are attached to the chromatids at the kinetochore. The chromatids separate and are pulled towards the centrioles. Once this step is completed the microtubules disaggregate, two new nuclear membranes form and the cell cleaves to produce two daughter cells.

A = False   This is a **monocyte**. **Basophils** have a bilobed nucleus that is usually obscured by the strongly basophilic cytoplasmic granules (as seen in a Giemsa-stained preparation such as this one). Monocytes, as seen here, have an indented or horseshoe-shaped nucleus. The cytoplasm is extensive and blue-grey in colour with smaller numbers of granules (see B below). Monocytes are the largest of the white blood cells (up to 20 μm in diameter) and constitute 2–10% of the total white cells.

B = True   Monocytes have two types of cytoplasmic granules. By electron microscopy, the granules are electron dense and surrounded by lipid membrane. Histochemical studies show that one type contains lysosomal enzymes and are lysosomes. The contents of the second granule type are as yet unclear. Monocytes are phagocytic cells that remove all types of debris and foreign materials from tissue. They migrate to sites of tissue damage and inflammation as well as patrolling almost every tissue in the body to sample and present antigenic material to **T lymphocytes**.

C = True   This is an **erythrocyte**, the anucleate cell whose major function is oxygen transport. Erythrocytes are devoid of cytoplasmic organelles and packed instead with **haemoglobin**. The lifespan of an erythrocyte is determined by the length of time it can maintain its unique **biconcave disc** shape. Maintenance of this shape requires energy to maintain ion gradients across the membrane. In the absence of mitochondria, the erythrocyte is dependent on anaerobic metabolism of glucose for energy. As there is no nucleus, the enzymes required for this process cannot be replaced, nor can the structural proteins that contribute to maintaining the shape of the erythrocyte. After approximately 120 days, these systems are degenerate, the erythrocyte is unable to maintain its shape and is removed from the circulation in the spleen.

D = True   Monocytes in the blood form part of the monocyte–macrophage system, the main scavenger system in the body. Other cells in this group are **Kupffer cells** in the liver, **Langerhans cells** of the skin, **dendritic cells** of lymphoid tissue, **microglia** of the central nervous system and **tissue macrophages** (**tissue histiocytes**). These cells scavenge and dispose of tissue debris, dead cells (e.g. old erythrocytes in the spleen) and are very prominent at sites of tissue necrosis or inflammation. The second, related function of these cells is presentation of processed antigen to T lymphocytes along with production of soluble factors (such as **interleukin 1** (**IL1**)) which are vital for production of an inflammatory and/or immune response.

E = True **Spectrin** is a major protein in the cytoskeleton of the red blood cells and is vital for maintaining the biconcave disc shape of these cells. The biconcave disc shape improves oxygen exchange approximately 20–30% in comparison to a spherical shape.

A = True This is **non-keratinising stratified squamous epithelium**, which is found at many sites in the body that are subjected to friction, such as the oropharynx, the oesophagus, and the vagina and cervix. The stratified squamous epithelium of the skin (the **epidermis**) has to withstand even greater frictional stress and has an additional layer of keratin on the surface.

B = False In normal stratified squamous epithelia, cell division takes place only in the basal layer, and thus **mitotic figures** (dividing cells) are only seen in this layer. The basal cells are compact and cuboidal in shape. As the daughter cells are pushed towards the surface, they mature into polygonal cells with plentiful cytoplasm which may be eosinophilic or may appear clear owing to its high glycogen content. As cells move further towards the surface, degeneration occurs with the nuclei becoming condensed and the entire cell becoming flattened. Eventually the cells loosen their connections with adjacent cells and break free from the surface (**desquamate**). These are the cells collected by the spatula or brush during the 'Pap smear test', a technique whereby the surface epithelial cells of the cervix may be examined for premalignant changes and frank malignancy.

C = True **Desmosomes** are present in great numbers in stratified squamous epithelia, and hold adjacent cells together. All epithelia have some desmosomes, however. The desmosomes are attached on their cytoplasmic face to the intermediate filaments of the epithelial cells.

D = False This, as mentioned above several times, is stratified squamous epithelium. **Transitional epithelium** is only found in the lower urinary tract. Stratified squamous epithelium has a surface layer of flattened epithelial cells, while the surface of transitional epithelium consists of **umbrella cells**, which give it a scalloped surface. Stratified squamous epithelium has cuboidal basal cells and large polygonal intermediate cells with plentiful cytoplasm. In transitional epithelium the basal and intermediate layer cells are similar to each other with less cytoplasm than intermediate layer squamous cells.

E = False Stratified squamous epithelium, like all other epithelia, contains **cytokeratin** intermediate filaments. **Desmin** intermediate filaments are characteristic of muscle tissue. The term cytokeratin actually describes a group of proteins of different molecular weights. Certain cytokeratin types are characteristic of certain epithelia. This fact can be very useful in diagnostic pathology where the presence of cytokeratins in a malignant tumour (as demonstrated by immunohistochemistry techniques) can identify that tumour as a *carcinoma* (i.e. derived from epithelial tissue). Other tumour types such as *sarcoma* (derived from supporting tissues) or *malignant melanoma* (derived from the *melanocytes* of the skin) contain different intermediate filaments or other cytoplasmic proteins characteristic of the cell of origin of the tumour. Furthermore, identification of different types of cytokeratin can help to further classify a *metastatic carcinoma* as likely to originate in certain organs.

PAPER 4 ANSWER 4.4

A = True Smooth muscle cells or fibres are arranged in groups known as *fasciculi*. The fibres of each fasciculus are arranged parallel to each other and each fasciculus forms a functional unit. The arrangement of the fasciculi varies from tissue to tissue. In this micrograph of *myometrium* (the smooth muscle wall of the uterus) the smooth muscle fasciculi are arranged in a random pattern.

B = False No *cross-striations* are found in smooth muscle in contrast to *skeletal* (*striated* or *voluntary*) *muscle* and *cardiac muscle*. Cross-striations, which appear as alternating fine dark and pale stripes in light micrographs, appear as a result of the regular arrangement of the myofibrils within the skeletal and cardiac muscle cells. In contrast, the contractile proteins of smooth muscle are arranged in a random fashion in the cells. The contractile proteins are anchored to *focal densities* (cytoplasmic) and *anchoring densities* (on the membranes).

C = False No branched fibres are found in smooth muscle. Smooth muscle cells are shaped like spindles, with tapering ends. In skeletal muscle, the muscle cells are larger than smooth muscle cells and are cylindrical in shape. Cardiac muscle cells are the only muscle cells that are branched. The ends of cardiac muscle cells abut each other and have complex intercellular junctions where the ends meet (*intercalated discs*).

D = True The nuclei are central in smooth muscle cells as can easily be seen in this micrograph. In skeletal muscle the nuclei are found at the margin of the cell and, because of the fusion of *myoblasts* during development, each fibre contains multiple nuclei. The nuclei of smooth muscle cells are 'cigar shaped', i.e. elongated with rounded (as opposed to pointed) ends. In cardiac muscle the nuclei are also centrally placed, but tend to be rounder and larger and binucleate cells are common.

E = True   The muscle fasciculi in this section are arranged randomly so that some nuclei are seen in transverse section and appear rounded, while others are cut in longitudinal section, showing their true elongated shape. This appearance is particularly prominent in the myometrium and bladder where the smooth muscle fascicles are randomly arranged. In the gastrointestinal tract the smooth muscle fasciculi are arranged into distinct layers (longitudinal and circular layers plus an oblique layer in the stomach) and within these layers the fasciculi are orientated parallel to each other.

PAPER 4   ANSWER 4.5

A = False   The cell nuclei within a nerve bundle or fascicle such as this one consist mainly of **Schwann cell** nuclei and the nucleus indicated probably belongs to a Schwann cell. Also scattered among the nerve fibres are occasional fibroblasts, the nuclei of which are more slender and elongated with more condensed chromatin than the Schwann cell nuclei. Nerve cell bodies (containing the nucleus) are not generally found within nerve fascicles but only in the central nervous system or in peripheral nerve ganglia. Nerve cell nuclei are easily identified by their large size, round shape and prominent nucleoli.

B = True   The **perineurium** is a condensed layer of collagenous supporting tissue that contains small numbers of fibroblasts, identifiable by their spindle-shaped nuclei. The dense collagen of the perineurium is continuous with the more delicate collagenous supporting tissue within the nerve fascicle, known as the **endoneurium**.

C = False   Peripheral nerves carry a mixture of autonomic and somatic nerve fibres. The two types of fibre cannot be distinguished on a routine H & E stained micrograph such as this one.

D = False   This nerve fascicle almost certainly consists of a mixture of **myelinated** and **non-myelinated** nerve fibres. Schwann cells surround both types of nerve fibre, forming the **myelin sheath** for myelinated fibres. Schwann cells, however, also envelope smaller nerve fibres within their cytoplasm and several fibres can be identified within the cytoplasm of a single Schwann cell (by electron microscopy). Autonomic nerve fibres and small sensory fibres of the peripheral nervous system are generally non-myelinated, while motor nerve fibres and larger sensory fibres are myelinated.

E = False   All peripheral nerves contain a mixture of **afferent** (sensory) and **efferent** (motor) somatic nerve fibres as well as autonomic nerve fibres.

A = False   **X** marks the ***tunica adventitia*** of the wall of this ***muscular artery***. The tunica adventitia, or simply the adventitia, is composed mainly of collagen and elastin, which is stained dark brown by this special stain which demonstrates elastic tissue.

B = True   Muscular arteries have two major layers of elastic tissue, the ***internal*** and ***external elastic laminae***. This is obviously the internal elastic lamina, which is thicker and better defined than the external elastic lamina.

C = False   As mentioned above, this is a muscular artery. ***Elastic arteries***, including the aorta, the innominate, carotid and subclavian arteries as well as the larger pulmonary vessels, have multiple layers of elastic tissue arranged concentrically in the ***tunica media***. The muscular arteries, with only two distinct layers of elastic tissue, include the coronary, cerebral, femoral, radial and renal arteries.

D = True   This is the tunica media, which consists of a layer of concentrically arranged smooth muscle cells. The thickness of the tunica media varies with the size of the vessels with smaller vessels having thinner media. The three layers of the walls of arteries include the ***tunica intima***, which is the delicate inner layer, the tunica media, and the outer tunica adventitia.

E = False   The tunica intima consists of a layer of flattened ***endothelial cells***. The underlying supporting tissue contains some elastic tissue as well as myointimal cells and fibroblasts. Accumulation of lipid in myointimal cells, probably following damage to the overlying endothelium, is one of the early events in the development of ***atheroma***, one of the leading causes of death in developed countries.

A = False   This is a ***merocrine*** or ***eccrine sweat gland*** of the skin. These glands are not associated with hair follicles but are scattered at random throughout the skin. The glands associated with hair follicles are the ***sebaceous glands***, which empty their secretions into the hair follicle. The sebaceous gland and hair follicle together make up the ***pilosebaceous unit***.

B = False   Merocrine sweat glands are found in the skin covering the whole body. ***Apocrine glands*** are restricted to the skin of the axillae, the genital aras and the areolae of the breast. Apocrine glands only become functional around puberty.

C = True   Merocrine glands secrete **sweat**, a watery fluid that is hypotonic
            with respect to plasma. As well as water, sweat contains sodium
            and chloride ions, which give it its salty taste, as well as other
            ions and small molecules like urea. Sweat serves to cool the
            body. Apocrine glands secrete a more viscid fluid, which is milky
            in colour. Sebaceous glands secrete **sebum**, which contains lipid.

D = True   The coiled **ducts** of the merocrine glands empty their secretions
            onto the skin surface via a sweat pore. The duct consists of two
            cell layers, the cells of which reabsorb sodium ions, making the
            sweat hypotonic. The unbranched coiled secretory part of the
            gland is lined by a single layer of cuboidal or columnar cells.
            These cells pump sodium ions into the lumen of the gland. Water
            molecules diffuse passively into the lumen in pursuit of the
            sodium ions.

E = False   **Decapitation secretion** is a feature of apocrine sweat glands.
            Sebaceous glands discharge their secretions by **holocrine
            secretion** whereby the entire cell is dissolved into the gland
            lumen, releasing its contents. The mechanism of secretion of
            merocrine glands, as described in D above, consists of active
            transport of sodium ions into the gland lumen followed by passive
            diffusion of water. In the duct some sodium ions are reabsorbed
            but because of lack of permeability of the epithelium to water, the
            water remains in the duct to be excreted on the skin surface.

PAPER 4   ANSWER 4.8

A = True   **Centres of ossification** arise in certain membranes during fetal
            development when **primitive mesenchymal cells** differentiate
            into **osteoblasts**. The osteoblasts secrete **osteoid**, forming
            centres of ossification. As the ossification centre enlarges,
            osteoblasts become trapped in the osteoid, become quiescent
            and are known as **osteocytes**. Osteocytes are just visible at this
            magnification as small dark dots within the bone.

B = True   The cells marked **Y** are osteoblasts. Plump osteoblasts can be
            seen surrounding the osteoid, while smaller osteocytes are
            embedded in the bone. Once the osteoid has been laid down,
            mineralisation proceeds by deposition of **hydroxyapatite
            crystals** in matrix vesicles. The matrix vesicles are formed by
            osteoblasts and consist of a surrounding membrane derived from
            osteoblast plasma membrane. The lumina of the matrix vesicles
            are filled with calcium and phosphate ions, which are the
            substrate for the formation of hydroxyapatite crystals.

C = False   **Intramembranous ossification** is typically seen in the flat bones
            of the skull. There is no framework of cartilage in this type of
            ossification. In contrast, most other bones in the developing fetus,

including long bones such as the femur and humerus, develop by ossification of hyaline cartilage known as ***endochondral ossification***.

D = True   When the ossification centres have enlarged and fused to form the skull bones, the resulting bone is cancellous bone with marrow spaces between the bony trabeculae. These spaces become colonised by ***haemopoietic cells*** and become active centres of blood cell production.

E = False   ***Epiphyseal growth plates*** (***epiphyses***) are a feature of long bones. These growth plates are found near the ends of the long bones. Bone growth, which is continuous throughout childhood, results from the deposition of cartilage that becomes progressively ossified. Bone growth ceases at puberty when the epiphyses fuse. In contrast, the flat bones of the skull are enlarged by the deposition of bone in the membrane at the edges of the bone plates. No epiphyseal growth plates are found in such bones.

PAPER 4   ANSWER 4.9

A = True   This is the ***white pulp*** of the spleen, which consists of organised lymphoid tissue. The white pulp of the spleen, like the organised lymphoid tissue of lymph nodes, Peyer's patches, and tonsils, is an organ of the immune defence system. In the spleen, as in other lymphoid organs, there are specific B and T lymphocyte areas. B lymphocytes are found as primary or secondary follicles, usually adjacent to a small arteriole. T lymphocytes are found arranged in a sheath surrounding the central arteries, an arrangement known as the ***periarteriolar lymphoid sheath*** or ***PALS***. Of course, as in other lymphoid tissues, a minor proportion of T cells are found in the B lymphocyte areas and vice versa.

B = True   The ***sheathed capillary*** is a structure unique to the red pulp of the spleen. Its function is to remove aged or damaged erythrocytes from the circulation. Sheathed capillaries are the terminal branches of ***penicillary arteries***. These small blind-ending vessels lack an endothelial lining but instead are lined by macrophages. Blood entering these vessels must pass through the macrophage barrier, traverse the ***cords of Bilroth*** (see C below) and enter the red pulp sinuses to return to the circulation. This is known as the ***open circulation model***.

C = False   The cords of Bilroth, along with the red pulp vascular sinuses, make up the ***red pulp*** of the spleen (marked **Y**). Erythrocytes leave the sheathed capillaries, which run in the cords of Bilroth, and pass through the parenchyma and the wall of the sinuses, to re-enter the circulation. The cords of Bilroth (the parenchyma) are packed with macrophages which phagocytose aged or abnormal red blood cells.

D = True   The lymphoid follicles of the spleen have a similar structure to those in other lymphoid tissue plus a well-defined outer zone of small lymphocytes known as the *marginal zone*. Thus the central pale *germinal centre* is surrounded by a *mantle zone* of small mature lymphocytes, which is in turn surrounded by a less closely packed zone of medium-sized lymphocytes, the marginal zone. Marginal zone lymphocytes display different surface markers than mantle zone lymphocytes and are thought to have different functions.

E = False   **Z** marks one of the trabeculae of the spleen. The trabeculae are continuous with the dense collagenous splenic capsule and extend into the parenchyma, providing structural support. In the trabecula marked **Z**, part of a moderate-sized vein can be seen. The trabeculae carry the larger vessels within the spleen. However, the spleen is not divided into well-defined lobes or lobules.

PAPER 4	ANSWER 4.10

A = False   The *thyroid gland* lies in close contact with the upper part of the *trachea* (not seen in this micrograph). However, it is clearly separate from it and does not extend into the wall of the trachea. These are submucosal *seromucinous glands*. The mucus secreted by these glands, along with the mucus from the *goblet cells* of the epithelium, helps to trap small particles in the inhaled air. The serous component of the secretions of these glands assists in humidifying the incoming air.

B = False   The cartilagenous rings of the trachea, along with the cartilage plates of the bronchi, consist of *hyaline cartilage*. Hyaline cartilage is relatively rigid yet elastic. It is also found in the nose, the ear, the costal cartilages and many joints. *Fibrocartilage* is found in the intervertebral discs and at other joints. The hyaline cartilage in the trachea is found as incomplete flattened circles, usually described as C-shaped. The opening of the ring is posterior and the two ends are bridged by the *trachealis muscle* (see below). The hyaline cartilage of the upper respiratory tree prevents collapse during inspiration.

C = False   The trachea is lined by *respiratory epithelium* from the level of the vocal cords to the level of the terminal bronchioles. The vocal cords, larynx and oropharynx are lined by stratified squamous epithelium. Respiratory epithelium is a *pseudostratified columnar epithelium* consisting of tall ciliated columnar cells, goblet cells, serous cells, Kulchitsky cells (neuroendocrine cells) and stem cells. The proportions of the different cell types are different at different levels of the trachea and at different levels of the respiratory tree.

D = True   The trachealis muscle, consisting of smooth muscle fibres, stretches across the gap between the ends of the hyaline cartilage rings. Contraction of the muscle reduces the diameter of the trachea during coughing. Relaxation of the trachealis allows elastic recoil of the cartilage rings to their maximum size.

E = True   The respiratory epithelium characteristically has a thick basement membrane.

PAPER 4   ANSWER 4.11

A = True   In the body of the stomach **parietal cells** are seen throughout the length of the glands but are most plentiful in the mid-portion. Parietal cells are easily recognised by their central rounded nucleus and plentiful eosinophilic (pink) cytoplasm. At this magnification they appear as pale pink dots clustered in the isthmus and neck of the gland. Parietal cells are the acid-secreting cells of the stomach. Their cytoplasm is packed with an extensive system of **canaliculi** and **tubulovesicular structures** that pump acid out of the cell into the lumen of the gland. They also secrete **intrinsic factor**.

B = False   This feature is found in the mucosa of the body and pyloric antrum and therefore does not discriminate between these two areas. The glands of the pyloric antrum, however, are branched and coiled in contrast to the straight glands of the gastric body. The glands of the pyloric antrum are lined throughout their length by mucus-secreting cells and lack parietal and **chief cells**.

C = False   **Paneth cells** are not found in either the gastric body or gastric antrum but characterise the mucosa of the small intestine crypts. Here they are found lining the bases of the crypts and can be identified by the collection of orange-red granules in the supranuclear cytoplasm.

D = True   The mucosa of the body of the stomach consists of straight tubular glands. In the pyloric antrum the glands are branched. In the body of the stomach from three to seven crypts empty into a single **gastric pit** or **foveola**.

E = False   Scattered **neuroendocrine cells**, which are almost impossible to identify in a low-power H&E photomicrograph, are situated in both the gastric body and pyloric antrum. They make up a small proportion of the total number of cells within the epithelial compartment. The major cells lining the bases of the crypts in the gastric body are **chief cells** (**peptic** or **zymogenic cells**). Chief cells secrete the enzyme **pepsin** and thus, in common with other protein-secreting cells, have large amounts of rough endoplasmic reticulum in their cytoplasm as well as membrane-bound secretory vesicles (**zymogen granules**).

A = False   The mucosa of the appendix has a similar structure to that of the colon except that lymphoid tissue is more prominent in the appendix. The glands or **crypts** are **straight simple glands** lined by simple columnar mucus-secreting epithelium. In contrast the mucosa of the ileum is arranged as tall **villi** with short crypts in between. The ileal epithelium consists of **enterocytes** with plentiful surface **microvilli**, interspersed with mucin-secreting goblet cells. **Paneth cells** with characteristic eosinophilic supranuclear granules are found in the bases of the crypts of the small intestinal mucosa.

B = False   Lymphoid tissue is prominent in the mucosa of the appendix at all ages but is generally more prominent in the young, becoming less conspicuous with age. The lymphoid tissue, which is part of the **gut-associated lymphoid tissue** (**GALT**) has a similar structure to **Peyer's patches** in the small intestine. Lymphoid follicles consisting of pale-staining **germinal centres** surrounded by a **mantle zone** are the main B cell area, while the interfollicular zones are packed with T cells.

C = False   Like the rest of the gastrointestinal tract the appendix has two layers of smooth muscle making up the **muscularis propria**. The inner layer, as elsewhere, is arranged circularly and the outer layer is arranged longitudinally. The exception to this general rule is the stomach, which has the same two layers of smooth muscle as well as an innermost oblique layer.

D = False   **Submucosal glands** are unnecessary in most of the gut as the mucosa produces enough mucin to lubricate the passage of the gut contents. The oesophagus and anus are lined by stratified squamous epithelium, which does not secrete mucin and therefore have submucosal glands for lubrication. In the duodenum, submucosal glands (**Brunner's glands**) produce an alkaline mucus that helps to neutralise the acidity of the **chyme** entering the duodenum from the stomach.

E = False   **Parietal cells** are found only in the stomach. These cells with round central nuclei and plentiful eosinophilic cytoplasm are responsible for the secretion of **gastric acid** and **intrinsic factor**. The majority of parietal cells are found in gastric body-type mucosa, which is found in the body and fundus of the stomach. Occasionally, however, a small number of parietal cells may be found in the gastric antrum.

A = False   Muscle fibres in the wall of the gall bladder are arranged in oblique, longitudinal and circumferential directions but there are no anatomically distinct layers. In this micrograph the muscle bundles are somewhat separated from each other by artefact occurring during preparation and this helps to demonstrate the random orientation of the bundles. This is unlike the rest of the gastrointestinal tract where there are distinct **inner circular** and **outer longitudinal layers**. The stomach, in addition, has an **inner oblique layer** so that the circular layer is the middle layer.

B = False   The lining of the gall bladder consists of a **simple columnar epithelium**. This is one of the few sites in the body where such an epithelium occurs. In most other sites columnar epithelia show various specialisations such as mucus secretion (colon, stomach, endocervix), or large numbers of surface microvilli as in the enterocytes of the small intestine.

C = True   As shown here, the **mucosa** has a folded configuration when not distended. However, the gall bladder can store up to about 100 ml of bile. In the distended state, the mucosa is flattened and the **submucosa**, which is loose and contains plentiful elastin fibres, is stretched.

D = False   I really hope that no-one thought this was true. Bile is of course secreted in the liver by **hepatocytes**. The bile passes into the **bile canaliculi** between the hepatocytes and thence through the **intrahepatic biliary tree** to the **right** and **left hepatic ducts** and the **common bile duct**. If the **sphincter of Oddi** at the lower end of the common bile duct is closed, bile passes along the **cystic duct** into the gall bladder. In the gall bladder the bile becomes concentrated as water is removed from the bile by the epithelium and passes into the submucosal lymphatics.

E = False   **Cholecystokinin-pancreozymin** (CCK) is the major stimulus to gall bladder contraction. CCK is secreted by **neuroendocrine cells** in the duodenal epithelium in response to the presence of chyme in the duodenum. CCK stimulates contraction of the muscle of the gall bladder wall. At the same time the sphincter of Oddi relaxes and bile flows along the cystic duct, the common bile duct and via the **ampulla of Vater** into the lumen of the duodenum where it emulsifies fats. **Glucagon** is secreted by the islets of Langerhans in the pancreas and raises blood glucose levels.

PAPER 4	ANSWER 4.14

A = True   The **renal corpuscle** is a spherical structure containing the **glomerulus**. The glomerulus is anchored to the surrounding structures by the **afferent** and **efferent arterioles**, which together make up the **vascular pole**. Opposite the vascular pole the **proximal convoluted tubule** joins the glomerulus to drain the ultrafiltrate of plasma produced by the glomerulus into the tubule.

The point where the proximal convoluted tubule joins the corpuscle is known as the **urinary pole**. In general, most of the renal corpuscles in a section of kidney will not be cut through the vascular and urinary poles as seen in this case.

B = True   **Bowman's capsule** is the layer of epithelium and its associated basement membrane that surrounds the glomerulus. Together Bowman's capsule and the glomerulus make up the renal corpuscle. Bowman's capsule encloses **Bowman's space**, which in life is filled with the ultrafiltrate of plasma produced by the glomerulus.

C = False   The cells that make up Bowman's capsule form a simple squamous epithelium, known as the **parietal layer** of Bowman's capsule. **Podocytes**, also sometimes known as the **visceral layer** of Bowman's capsule, are the epithelial cells that invest the outer surface of the glomerular capillaries. The visceral and parietal layers of Bowman's capsule are continuous with each other and the arrangement is reminiscent of the two layers of pleura lining the lungs. The podocytes are highly specialised cells, which form a major component of the glomerular filtration mechanism. They are named podocytes because each cell has numerous processes that branch to form the **pedicels** or **foot processes** that cover the outer surface of the **glomerular basement membrane**. The foot processes interdigitate with each other leaving slit-like spaces between them.

D = True   The **mesangial cells** and their product **mesangial matrix** form the specialised supporting tissue of glomerular capillary loops. Mesangial matrix has a similar chemical structure to basement membrane. Mesangial cells, in addition to producing matrix, have a number of other functions including phagocytosis and secretion of vasoactive substances. They also contain actin and myosin filaments and are contractile. Mesangial cells are thus able to control the flow of blood in the glomerular capillaries.

E = True   The endothelium of the glomerular capillary loops, together with the glomerular basement membrane and the podocytes, constitute the mechanism that filters plasma to form an ultrafiltrate, which is the first step in the formation of urine. These endothelial cells have large numbers of larger-than-usual fenestrations measuring 70–100 nm in diameter. Unlike fenestrated endothelium elsewhere in the body, the fenestrations do not have a diaphragm.

A = True   These cells are **chief** or **principal cells**. These are the main secretory cells of the parathyroid gland. They have a round central nucleus and cytoplasm which is either palely eosinophilic or clear on an H. & E stain. The variable staining is dependent on whether the cells are actively synthesising **parathormone** (**PTH**) or not. Actively secreting cells have plentiful rER in the cytoplasm and therefore stain with eosin (eosinophilic). Inactive cells have less rER and the cytoplasm is pale or clear.

B = False   The tissue marked **Y** is **adipose tissue**, which is a normal component of parathyroid glands in adults. The amount of adipose tissue present is quite variable but constitutes 25–40% of the total parathyroid. In the elderly the proportion of adipose tissue in the gland increases.

C = False   The cells marked **X** are chief or principal cells (see A above). Normal adult glands also contain nodules or clusters of **oxyphil cells** (marked **Z**).

D = True   These cells are oxyphil cells, which as mentioned above form nodules or clusters in normal parathyroids in young people as well as in the elderly. In H & E sections, these cells can be distinguished from chief cells by their copious eosinophilic cytoplasm. The appearance of the cytoplasm is due to its being packed with mitochondria. These cells do not secrete PTH and therefore do not contribute to the activity of the gland. Oxyphil cells increase in number with age.

E = True   The usual number of parathyroid glands in normal individuals is four, arranged as two pairs near the posterior surface of the thyroid gland. However five or six parathyroids may be found in a small proportion of asymptomatic individuals, making life difficult for the surgeon who is carrying out a parathyroidectomy (e.g. in individuals with **parathyroid hyperplasia**). The parathyroids are also notorious for their variable position in the neck, occasionally being found in the mediastinum and not uncommonly embedded in the thyroid gland.

PAPER 4	ANSWER 4.16

A = False   In a **seminiferous tubule** there is greater stratification of the cells lining the tubule, with plentiful mitotic figures. **Spermatozoa** will usually be visible within the lumen of a seminiferous tubule. Spermatozoa are often seen within the epididymis also but none are visible in this micrograph. The cell types in a seminiferous tubule include the various stages of germ cell development as well as **Sertoli cells**.

B = True   The **epididymal tubules** are lined by a tall columnar pseudostratified epithelium. These cells have long microvilli, incorrectly named as **stereocilia**.

C = False   The **prostatic urethra** is lined by transitional epithelium. The more distal part of the male urethra is lined by pseudostratified or stratified columnar epithelium.

D = False   The **rete testis** is lined by a simple cuboidal epithelium with much shorter microvilli plus a single **flagellum** on each cell.

E = False   The band of cells surrounding this tubule is made up of smooth muscle cells. The presence of a defined band of smooth muscle identifies this tubule as the more distal part of the epididymis.

A = False   These cells are **endometrial stromal cells**, which have become **decidualised**. When fertilisation and implantation occur, the increased progesterone levels cause proliferation and enlargement of endometrial stromal cells. These cells now have greatly increased cytoplasm which appears eosinophilic (pink) owing to the presence of numerous mitochondria and intermediate filaments. **Syncytiotrophoblast cells** are multinucleated cells derived from the placenta. These cells, along with **intermediate trophoblast cells**, infiltrate the endometrium where they penetrate into maternal vessels to allow maternal blood to circulate through the lacunae of the placenta. No syncytiotrophoblast cells are seen in this micrograph and although intermediate trophoblast cells are probably present they cannot be identified at this magnification.

B = False   This structure is a dilated **endometrial gland**, which is filled with secretions (mainly glycogen).

C = False   Endometrial stromal cells do not synthesise sex hormones. These cells respond to hormones during the course of the **menstrual cycle** and during pregnancy. The major source of progestagens in early pregnancy is the **corpus luteum of pregnancy**, found in the ovary. The **luteinised granulosa cells** of the corpus luteum of pregnancy secrete progestagens to maintain the pregnancy until the placenta is well enough developed (after about the third month) to take over the secretion of oestrogens and progestagens.

D = False   The appearance of **decidualised endometrium** infiltrated by trophoblast cells is seen only in pregnancy. Decidualisation of the stromal cells without trophoblast may, however, occur. There is often mild decidualisation in the late secretory phase of a normal menstrual cycle and decidualisation may also occur in individuals taking hormones for therapeutic reasons, e.g. hormone replacement therapy in postmenopausal women and in women taking the contraceptive pill.

E = False   This is a dilated capillary. The **spiral arteries**, which are prominent in the late secretory phase of the cycle, have a much smaller diameter in relation to their wall thickness. As they have a spiral shape, a section through the endometrium will show several profiles of a single artery. Dilated vessels are a common feature of decidualised endometrium.

A = False   This is a **terminal branch** of the breast ductal system. The **lactiferous ducts** are the large ducts that drain each lobe of the breast (15–25 in all) onto the surface of the nipple. Lactiferous ducts are therefore found only in the tissue deep to the nipple and are not associated with acini.

B = True   The **terminal duct–lobular unit** (**TDLU**) is the milk-producing component of breast tissue. Each consists of a terminal duct (**X**) plus a **lobule** made up of multiple **acini**, embedded in collagenous supporting tissue.

C = True   The epithelium of the breast ducts and lobules consists of two cell layers, a luminal layer of tall columnar secretory cells and a partial basal layer of **myoepithelial cells** (see D below).

D = True   The deeper basal cell layer of the breast epithelium is an incomplete layer of cells that show some characteristics of epithelial cells and some features of muscle cells, including the presence of **actin filaments**. These **myoepithelial cells** are stellate in shape and contract during lactation to move the secreted milk along the duct.

E = True   During pregnancy there is a marked proliferation of epithelial cells of the terminal ducts to increase the numbers of secretory acini. The acini also enlarge in size. Thus at the end of pregnancy and during lactation, the breast tissue consists largely of TDLUs in contrast with non-pregnant, non-lactating breast, which consists mainly of fibrous and adipose supporting tissue.

A = True   The **rods** and **cones** are the photoreceptor cells of the retina. These cells convert incoming light into nerve impulses by means of their content of visual pigments and unique membrane system. The cell bodies are in the deepest of the three cellular layers of the retina. The other two cellular layers include the **inner nuclear layer** and the **ganglion cell layer**. The ganglion cell layer is the cellular layer closest to the surface and contains cell bodies of the neurones that carry the nerve impulses to the brain. The cellular layer between these two, the inner nuclear layer, contains the cell bodies of interconnecting neurones that synapse with the other two cell layers.

B = False   The most superficial layer of the retina, which contains the optic nerve fibres, is separated from the vitreous body by the **inner limiting membrane** (not identifiable at this magnification). No epithelial cells are found here. The only epithelial cells in the retina are the pigmented epithelial cells in the deepest layer.

C = False   This is the **inner plexiform layer**. No blood vessels are found in the deep layers of the retina. Branches of the central artery of the retina run in the most superficial layer of the retina, the optic nerve fibre layer, and the superficial layers are dependent on diffusion from these vessels. Likewise the outer layers receive oxygen and nutrients by diffusion from the blood supply of the **choroid**.

D = True   **Müller cells**, which are long, ribbon-like cells, are found in most of the layers of the retina, extending through almost its full thickness. These cells perform support functions and are equivalent to the neuroglial cells found in the central nervous system. Intercellular junctions between rods and cones on the one hand and Müller cells on the other, form the inaccurately named '**outer limiting membrane**' of the retina.

E = True   Nerve impulses generated by incident light on the rods and cones pass to the interconnecting neurones of the inner nuclear layer (**bipolar cells**, **amacrine cells** and **horizontal cells**). These cells form multiple synapses with rods and cones and with the nerve cells of the innermost ganglion cell layer, which contains the cell bodies of the optic tract neurones. The layer marked **Y** contains the axons of these nerve cells passing towards the optic disc. Here the axons pass through the sclera and are carried in the optic nerve to the brain.

PAPER 4   ANSWER 4.20

A = False   The saw-tooth pattern of the endometrial glands seen here is the classic appearance of the late **secretory phase** of the cycle. At this stage the glands appear slightly dilated and the lumina are usually full of secretions. The saw-tooth appearance is due to the coiling of the glands and also the ragged nature of the epithelium, which has discharged its secretions. In the early **proliferative phase**, the endometrial glands are much more sparse, shorter and generally straight. As the proliferative phase progresses, the glands become elongated and eventually coiled. The saw-tooth appearance seen here is not seen in the proliferative phase.

B = False   The **endometrial stroma** consists of ovoid cells, which change in appearance greatly throughout the menstrual cycle. These cells are not smooth muscle cells, nor epithelial cells. Smooth muscle cells make up the **myometrium**, which is just seen in the lower part of this micrograph. You will note that the interface between myometrium and endometrium is irregular and rather ragged. This is an important point for the diagnostic pathologist trying to assess whether **endometrial carcinoma** has invaded into the myometrium of the uterus.

C = True **Spiral arterioles** are a prominent feature of the stroma in the late secretory phase of the cycle. This micrograph is rather too low-power for easy identification of spiral arterioles. These arterioles, however, can be identified at higher power by the multiple cross-sections of arteriole found close together. This is due to the coiling of the arterioles, so that a section through them cuts through several profiles of the same arteriole. The spiral arterioles begin to contract during the late secretory phase. This leads to ischaemia of the most superficial parts of the endometrium (the **stratum spongiosum** and **stratum compactum**), which are shed as menses. The deepest layer of the endometrium, the **stratum basalis**, does not contain spiral arterioles and is not lost during menstruation.

D = False Secretions are only found within the **luteal phase** of the cycle, which is equivalent to the secretory phase of the endometrium. The **follicular phase** of the cycle equates to the proliferative phase of the endometrial cycle. Secretions are only seen in the glands in the second half (luteal or secretory) of the cycle when ovulation has occurred.

E = False The lower part of the endometrium, the stratum basalis, does not change its appearance during the course of the menstrual cycle the way the upper layers change. The stratum basalis does not respond to ovulation and enter the secretory phase. No spiral arterioles are present in the stratum basalis so that this layer is not shed during menstruation and remains as the reserve layer for reconstitution of the endometrium at the end of menstruation.

A = True **X** is a **mitochondrion**. These are easily recognisable, even at low power, because of their inner folded membrane and outer smooth membrane. The folds of the inner membrane are known as **cristae**, giving the interior a striped appearance. Mitochondria vary in shape, but are generally ovoid. However, when seen in cross-section as several mitochondria are in this micrograph they can appear to be round. Mitochondria are the source of energy production of the cell, performing many of the functions of **cellular respiration**. The complex membrane system of the mitochondrion, plus the matrix, contains many of the enzymes of **Krebs' cycle**.

B = True The cytoplasm of this cell is indeed packed with **rough endoplasmic reticulum (rER)**. Rough endoplasmic reticulum consists of flattened cisternae of lipid membrane with ribosomes dotted over the surface. At this magnification the ribosomes appear as fine dots on the surface of the lipid membranes. Ribosomes synthesise proteins using **messenger RNA (mRNA)** as a template for the protein sequence. Protein synthesised by ribosomes on the surface of rER is inserted into the lumen of the rER where further processing takes place. Proteins are then transported within membrane-bound vesicles to the Golgi apparatus for further modification, and thence to the cell surface for secretion by *exocytosis*. The large amount of rER in the cytoplasm of this cell is characteristic of cells specialised for protein production and secretion.

C = True   **Y** is the nuclear membrane, which is made up of two lipid bilayers. The basic lipid *bilayer membrane* consists of two layers of phospholipids, arranged in such a way that the hydrophobic tails are towards the centre, with the hydrophilic heads on the outer surface. This is the basic structure of the *plasma membrane*, which surrounds the cytoplasm, and the membranes which make up the rER and *smooth endoplasmic reticulum (sER)*. The nucleus is surrounded by two such membranes, the outer of which is continuous with the rER and sER. As well as phospholipids, all membranes include intrinsic proteins, carbohydrates and cholesterol.

D = True   The double layer of the nuclear membrane is interrupted by *nuclear pores*. These are gaps in the membrane, which are lined by complex protein structures. These gaps allow large molecules of RNA to move from the nucleus to the cytoplasm. They probably also perform a function in holding the two lipid membranes together.

E = False   The structure marked **Z** is the *Golgi apparatus*. This is the site where proteins synthesised in the rER are modified by the addition of carbohydrate molecules and then packaged into transport vesicles for excretion at the surface of the cell. The Golgi apparatus is composed of flattened cisternae of lipid membrane arranged in a saucer-shaped, or concave, stack, with the concave face of the stack facing towards the nucleus. In general the Golgi apparatus is found close to the nucleus. Cells with high protein production may contain several Golgi apparati.

PAPER 4	ANSWER 4.22

A = False   These fibres have the characteristic appearance of *type I collagen*. They are arranged as parallel fibres with the typical *cross-banding pattern*. This is not seen in collagen type IV, which forms a mesh structure and is a major component of basement membranes. Collagen type I has great tensile strength and is very widespread in many tissues including the dermis of the skin, tendons and ligaments.

B = True   Collagen is secreted into the *extracellular matrix* in the form of *tropocollagen*. Each tropocollagen molecule consists of three identical polypeptide chains, known as *alpha chains*. The alpha chains are coiled together to form a helix measuring 300 nm in length and 1.5 nm in diameter. In the extracellular environment the tropocollagen molecules polymerize to form collagen fibrils.

C = True   The polymerization of tropocollagen molecules occurs in an orderly fashion giving rise to the cross-banding pattern which is well demonstrated here. Contrast this pattern with the structure of skeletal muscle and it can be seen that the two are quite different although the novice electron microscopist may find this confusing. The cross-banding of collagen cannot be seen at the magnifications achieved by light microscopy and is only visible by electron microscopy. High-power light microscopy, however, can demonstrate the banding pattern of skeletal muscle, using appropriate staining methods. At the top of this micrograph there are a few collagen fibres cut in transverse section, appearing as solid round structures. The cross-banded pattern cannot be seen in this view.

D = False   Collagen and most of the other components of extracellular matrix are secreted by **fibroblasts**. Fibroblasts are cells derived from the mesenchyme of the embryo. They are extremely widespread throughout the body and are seen in most tissues as spindle-shaped nuclei with fairly scanty cytoplasm. **Macrophages**, which are also derived from mesenchyme precursors, belong to the haemopoietic series of cells. Macrophages are motile cells which wander the body engulfing debris and regulating the immune response via the presentation of antibody to lymphocytes and secretion of regulatory factors. Macrophages are also extremely widespread throughout the body and are recognisable by their kidney-shaped nuclei and plentiful faintly staining cytoplasm. The cytoplasm of macrophages may be foamy in appearance owing to phagocytosis of extracellular material.

E = False   As mentioned above, collagen type I is prominent in many supporting tissues, especially those requiring great tensile strength. **Type II collagen** is the main collagen found in hyaline cartilage. Type II collagen does not have a cross-banding pattern because the fine fibrils are dispersed in a meshwork through the ground substance.

PAPER 4   ANSWER 4.23

A = False   This is the cell nucleus and is composed entirely of **euchromatin**. Euchromatin consists of chromosomes that are not tightly coiled but rather are dispersed throughout the nucleus. This generally indicates that active RNA synthesis is going on, as RNA synthesis can only take place in uncoiled chromosomes. Areas of euchromatin by light microscopy appear paler and less haematoxyphilic (blue). Heterochromatin consists of tightly coiled chromosomes that appear more haematoxyphilic by light microscopy.

B = True   The nucleus is surrounded by the ***nuclear envelope***, which consists of two bilayered lipid membranes closely apposed to each other. The nuclear envelope cannot be resolved into two layers at this magnification but it can be seen around the periphery of the nucleus. The two layers of the nuclear envelope are penetrated by plentiful ***nuclear pores***, which allow the passage of RNA and proteins between the nucleus and the cytoplasm. Nuclear pores are protein structures which as well as maintaining an opening in the nuclear membrane, probably also hold the two lipid bilayers together somewhat in the manner of rivets.

C = True   **Y** indicates the ***nucleolus***. Ganglion cells characteristically have a prominent nucleolus. The nucleolus is the site of synthesis of ***ribosomal RNA*** (***rRNA***). The rRNA is synthesised in the nucleolus and also assembled into ribosomes there. Assembly of ribosomes involves the incorporation of proteins (many of which are enzymes) into the ribosomal structure. The ribosomal proteins are of course synthesised in the cytoplasm as are all other cell proteins (see E below).

D = False   ***Histone proteins*** are an important component of the nuclear protein. The nucleus consists of approximately 20% DNA, the rest of its substance being made up of nuclear protein and RNA. Histone proteins are one type of nuclear protein, the remainder being called ***non-histone proteins***. Histone proteins bind tightly to DNA and are important in controlling the coiling of the DNA strand. They are thus integral structural components of chromosomes. Non-histone proteins include all the other protein types found in the nucleus, including enzymes and regulatory proteins.

E = False   Protein synthesis occurs in the cytoplasm only. ***Messenger RNA*** (***mRNA***) is synthesised from the DNA template within the nucleus. The strand of mRNA is then transported through the nuclear pores into the cytoplasm where it links to one or more ribosomes. The ribosomes use the 'recipe' for protein structure indicated by the sequence of ***codons*** of the mRNA to synthesise the required protein. Protein synthesis may take place either on free ribosomes within the cytoplasm or ribosomes bound to rER. Most of the proteins synthesised on rough endoplasmic reticulum are destined either for incorporation into a membrane (the plasma membrane of the cell, lysosomal membranes) or for secretion into the extracellular space. Proteins that are destined for the nucleus such as histone and non-histone proteins and the proteins required for ribosomes are then transported back through the nuclear pores into the nucleus. Ribosomal RNA as mentioned above is synthesised in the nucleolus, probably in the area known as the ***filamentous component*** of the nucleolus. Assembly of rRNA and ribosomal proteins into ribosome subunits is thought to take place in the paler ***granular component*** of the nucleolus. In this micrograph, the granular and filamentous components are not easily identified.

A = True   **X** marks the nucleus of an ***endothelial cell***. Endothelial cells are flattened and line the blood vessel with a thin layer of cytoplasm that can easily be seen around the rest of the capillary. The nucleus bulges into the lumen of the capillary, where it can just be resolved by light microscopy. The thin layer of cytoplasm surrounding the rest of the capillary is not usually visible with the light microscope.

B = True   Where the plasma membranes of adjacent endothelial cells (or indeed a single endothelial cell) meet, they form a tight junction of the ***fascia occludens*** type. These junctions prevent leakage of the capillary contents through the wall of the capillary. The opposing cell membranes are very closely apposed to each other and in some areas the plasma membranes appear to fuse completely. At very high-power electron microscopy, a system of fine matching ridges can be seen between the two layers of plasma membrane. Characteristic of capillary endothelium is a small cytoplasmic flap, known as a ***marginal fold***, which extends from one endothelial cell, over the adjacent cell, and indeed such a marginal flap can be seen in this micrograph.

C = False   **Z** marks a very thin layer of ***pericyte*** cytoplasm. Capillaries contain no smooth muscle in their walls, the walls consisting of endothelial cells and their basement membranes. On the outer side of the capillary wall there is a discontinuous layer of pericytes. In this micrograph, only the pericyte cytoplasm is seen. The nucleus is not included in this plane of section. The pericyte also has its own basement membrane, which cannot be seen at this magnification. Pericytes are thought to have some contractile function. Note the scattered strands of collagen around the periphery of the pericyte, which form part of the supporting tissue. Note that there has been some separation of the tissues in this micrograph, during preparation.

D = False   Endothelial cells have many metabolic functions in addition to their function as a permeability barrier. Endothelial cells produce the ***collagen*** and ***proteoglycans*** which make up their basement membrane. They also synthesise and secrete some of the factors of the coagulation cascade, e.g. ***Von Willebrand factor***, as well as various factors which minimise unwanted thrombus formation such as ***thrombomodulin*** and ***nitrous oxide***. Endothelial cells secrete vasoactive factors and molecules which mediate acute inflammation. These factors include ***prostacyclin***, ***endothelin*** and ***interleukins 1***, ***6*** and ***8***. Endothelial cells have also been shown to produce some growth factors such as ***fibroblast growth factor***.

E = False   ***Birbeck granules*** are characteristic of ***Langerhans cells***. Langerhans cells are part of the monocyte–macrophage system

189

and are thought to function as antigen-presenting cells in the skin. Endothelial cells have a cytoplasmic membrane-bound organelle, known as the **_Weibel–Palade body_** that stores Von Willebrand factor (factor VIII in the coagulation cascade). This micrograph has not high enough magnification to demonstrate the Weibel–Palade bodies.

PAPER 5

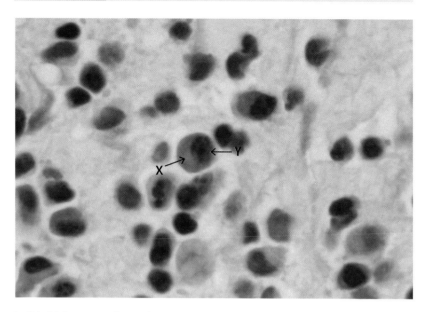

In this high-power photomicrograph of a plasma cell stained by the routine H & E method:

A The amphophilic (purple) colour of the cytoplasm is due to the presence of plentiful mitochondria.

B The area marked **X** indicates the Golgi apparatus.

C The nucleus contains euchromatin.

D The structure marked **Y** is the site of antibody synthesis.

E Immunoglobulins for export are found free in the cytoplasm.

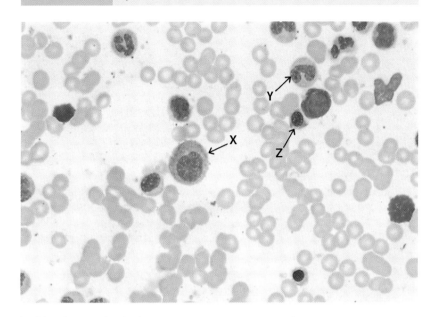

In this micrograph of a bone marrow smear:

A   The cell marked **X** is a myelocyte.

B   The cell marked **Y** is an osteoclast.

C   The cell marked **X** contains haemoglobin.

D   The cell marked **Z** will extrude its nucleus before becoming a mature cell.

E   Azurophilic granules are found in the cell marked **Z**.

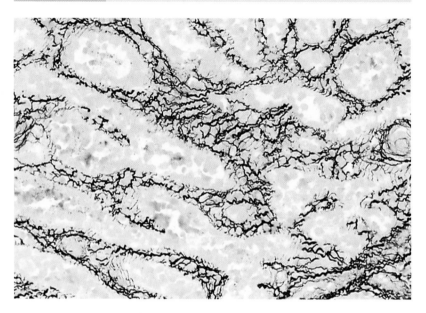

This micrograph of spleen is stained by a special method to demonstrate reticulin:

A   The black-stained fibrous components consist of collagen type III.

B   These fibres are easily identified in H & E stained sections.

C   The black components are also found in abundance in the liver.

D   By electron microscopy, the black components would have a cross-banding pattern.

E   The black fibres are anchored to the capsule of the spleen.

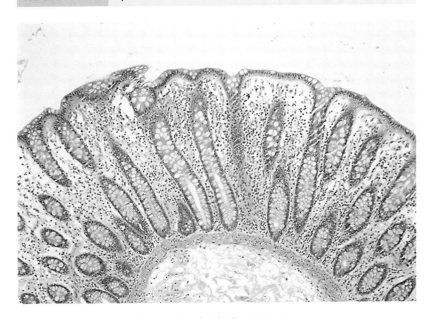

In this medium-power micrograph of colonic mucosa:

A   The epithelium is of simple columnar type.

B   The glands are compound acinar type.

C   The epithelial cells have clear cytoplasm owing to their content of glycogen.

D   The epithelial cells are attached to the basement membrane by junctional complexes.

E   Neuroendocrine cells are scattered through the epithelium.

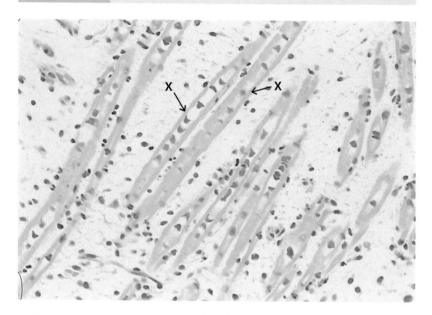

In this micrograph of developing fetal skeletal muscle:

A   The cells marked **X** are myoblasts.

B   At maturity the cell nuclei will be found at the periphery of the cell.

C   The contractile proteins are already fully formed at this stage of development.

D   The cells contain plentiful mRNA for the protein myosin.

E   These cells are formed by fusion of more primitive precursor cells.

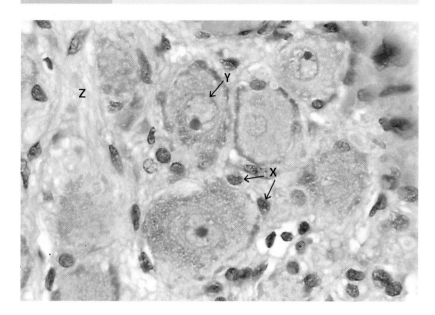

In this high-power photomicrograph of peripheral nerve tissue:

A The cells identified by **X** are oligodendrocytes.

B The brown pigment within the cytoplasm of the large cells identifies this tissue as part of the substantia nigra.

C The structure marked **Y** is a nerve cell nucleus.

D The brown pigment is melanin.

E The area marked **Z** contains plentiful axons and dendrites.

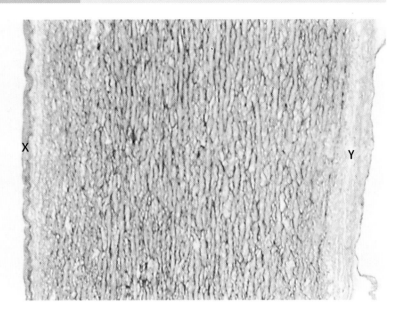

This micrograph is of an artery stained by a special method for elastin:

A   It could be the common carotid artery.

B   It could be the radial artery.

C   The structure marked **X** is the tunica intima.

D   The structure marked **Y** contains vasa vasorum.

E   There is no smooth muscle in the tunica media.

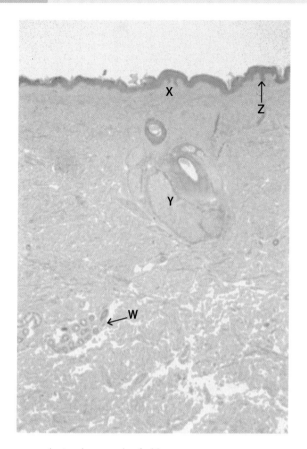

In this low-power photomicrograph of skin:

A   The area marked **X** is the reticular dermis.

B   The structure marked **Y** is an eccrine (merocrine) sweat gland.

C   The structure marked **Z** is a rete ridge.

D   The cutaneous vascular plexus is found in the upper part of the dermis.

E   Secretion in the gland marked **W** is by decapitation of the secretory cells.

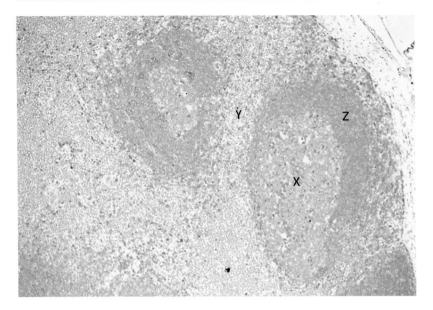

This is a medium-power micrograph of lymph node, stained by the immunoperoxidase method using an antibody that binds to B lymphocytes, thus staining them brown. The capsule of the lymph node can be seen at the upper right corner of the micrograph, and:

A   The structure marked **X** is a germinal centre.

B   **Y** marks the medulla of the lymph node.

C   **X** is composed entirely of B lymphocytes and supporting tissue.

D   **Z** is called the marginal zone.

E   High endothelial venules are found in the area marked **Y**.

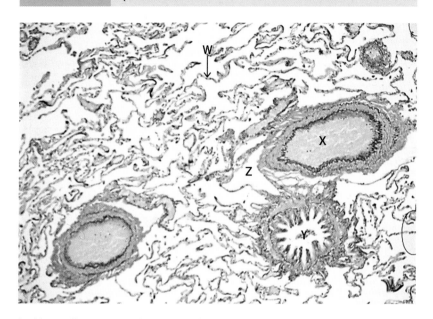

In this medium-power micrograph of lung stained by a special method to demonstrate elastin:

A   The structure marked **X** is a branch of the pulmonary artery.

B   The structure marked **Y** is a segmental bronchus.

C   The space marked **Z** would be filled with blood during life.

D   The structure **W** is lined on both sides mainly by type I pneumocytes.

E   the wall of the structure marked **X** is composed mainly of smooth muscle and elastin fibres.

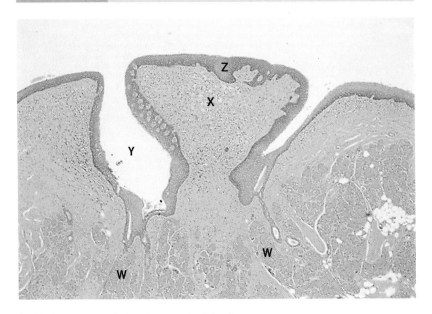

In this low-power photomicrograph of the tongue:

A   The structure marked **X** is a filiform papilla.

B   The taste buds are found scattered in the epithelium lining the clefts **Y**.

C   The structure marked **X** is found only in the anterior one-third of the tongue.

D   The epithelium marked **Z** is a pseudostratified columnar type epithelium.

E   The structure marked **W** is a mucous gland.

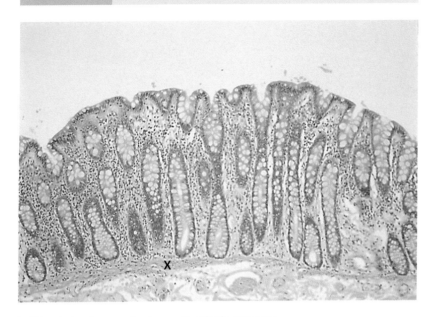

In this photomicrograph of normal colonic mucosa:

A   The epithelium is composed mainly of enterocytes.

B   Plasma cells are prominent in the lamina propria.

C   The muscularis propria is seen at the lower part of the micrograph (labelled **X**).

D   The crypts are branched tubular glands.

E   A major function of the epithelial cells is the absorption of water.

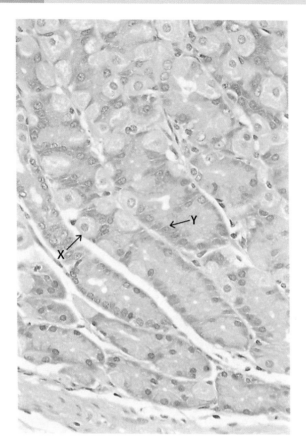

In this high-power micrograph of the base of a gland from the body of the stomach:

A   The cell marked **X** has an extensive cytoplasmic canalicular membrane system.

B   The cell marked **Y** secretes intrinsic factor.

C   The cell marked **X** secretes gastrin.

D   The cell marked **Y** secretes mucin.

E   The cell marked **X** acts as a reserve cell.

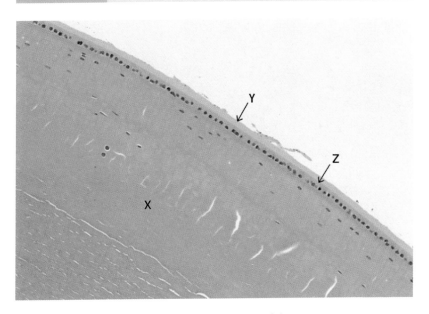

In this high-magnification micrograph of the lens of the eye:

A   The area marked **X** consists of fibres packed with crystallins.

B   The shape of the lens is altered by contraction of the smooth muscle of the ciliary body.

C   The structure marked **Y** is the lens capsule.

D   The cells marked **Z** make up the posterior cuboidal epithelium.

E   The lens is derived from mesoderm in the embryo.

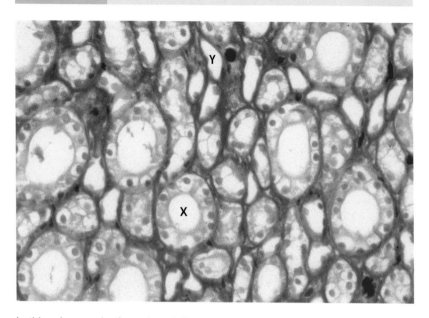

In this micrograph of renal medulla:

A   The structure marked **X** is a collecting duct.

B   The structure marked **Y** is a thin limb of the loop of Henle.

C   The structure marked **X** is responsive to antidiuretic hormone.

D   The interstitium has a high concentration of urea.

E   The structure marked **Y** actively transports sodium ions into the interstitium.

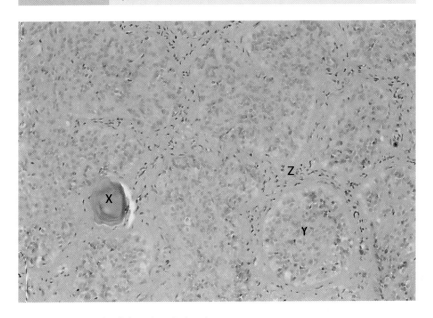

In this micrograph of the pineal gland:

A   The structure marked **X** contains calcium.

B   The cells of the structure marked **Y** secrete the hormone melatonin.

C   The cells of the structure marked **Y** respond to light and darkness.

D   The cells in the area marked **Z** are fibroblasts.

E   The cells marked **Y** probably regulate immune functions.

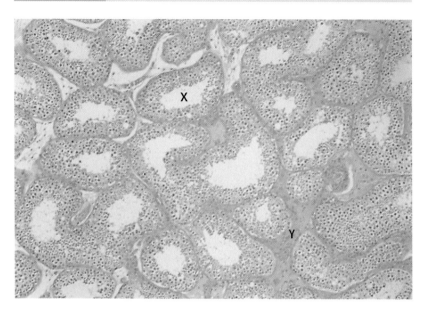

In this medium-power photomicrograph of testis:

A   The structure marked **X** is the site of production of male gametes.

B   The structure marked **X** contains Leydig cells within its basement membrane.

C   For each spermatid produced, three degenerate polar bodies are also produced.

D   The structure marked **X** has a wall consisting of two layers of smooth muscle cells.

E   Cells in the area marked **Y** secrete testosterone.

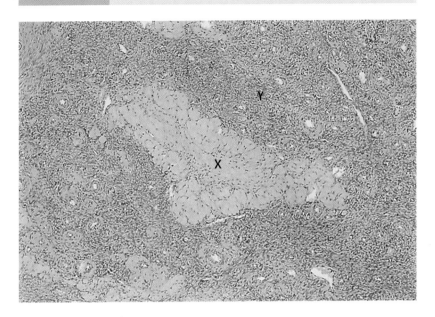

In this micrograph of ovary:

A   The structure marked **X** is a corpus luteum.

B   The cells indicated by **Y** are identical to the stromal cells of the endometrium.

C   The functions of the cells indicated by **Y** include secretion of hormones.

D   The structure marked **X** persists for life.

E   The production of ova takes place in the structure marked **X**.

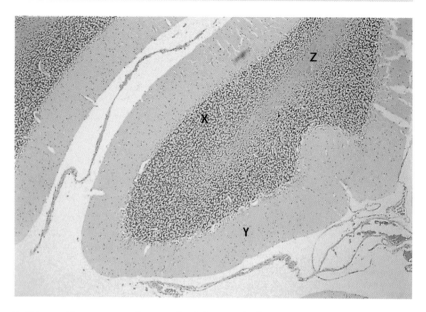

In this medium-power micrograph of the cerebellum:

A   The structure marked **X** is the granular layer.

B   The structure marked **Y** contains plentiful neurones.

C   Purkinje cells are found at the junction of **X** and **Y**.

D   The structure marked **Z** contains mainly unmyelinated neurones.

E   Golgi cells are found in the structure marked **Y**.

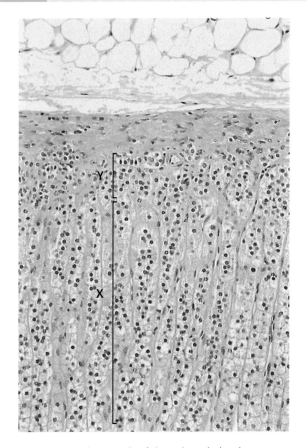

In this high-power photomicrograph of the adrenal gland:

A The cells in the area marked **X** are arranged in clusters.

B The area marked **Y** is the zona reticularis.

C Adrenaline is secreted by the cells in the area marked **Y**.

D The cells in the area marked **X** contain plentiful smooth endoplasmic reticulum.

E The area marked **Y** receives its blood supply from the short cortical arteries.

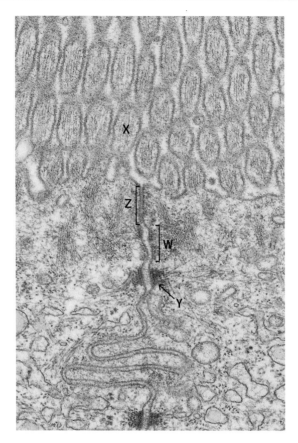

In this high-magnification electron micrograph of the epithelium of the small bowel:

A The structure marked **X** is a microvillus.

B The structure marked **Y** is a tight junction.

C The function of the structure marked **Z** is to attach the cells to each other.

D Similar structures to **Y** are found at the base of the epithelium.

E The structure marked **W** is a zonula adherens.

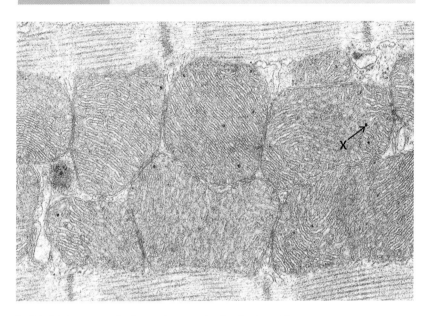

In this high-power electron micrograph of mitochondria:

A   The outer membrane contains porin.

B   The structure marked **X** is a matrix granule.

C   Many of the enzymes of Krebs' cycle are found within the matrix.

D   The mitochondria are surrounded by free ribosomes.

E   Mitochondria contain DNA.

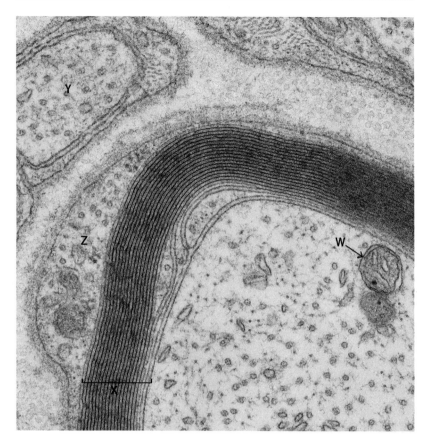

In this high-magnification lateral micrograph of peripheral nerve cut in transverse section:

A   **X** marks the myelin sheath.

B   **Y** marks a non-myelinated axon.

C   The Schwann cell cytoplasm is marked by **Z**.

D   The axons contain microtubules.

E   The structure marked **W** is part of the cell nucleus.

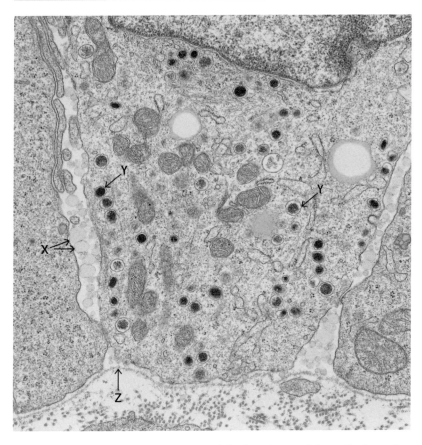

In this high-power electron micrograph of the basal part of the epithelium of the small bowel:

A   The structures marked **X** contain lipid.

B   The structures marked **Y** are dense core granules.

C   The cell containing **Y** has plentiful surface microvilli.

D   The structures marked **X** pass from the lumen of the small bowel directly into the intercellular space.

E   The structure marked **Z** is the basement membrane of the epithelium.

A = False   The cytoplasm of plasma cells stains a characteristic *amphophilic* or purple colour by the H & E method because of the presence of plentiful RNA and protein in the cytoplasm. RNA is *basophilic*, staining strongly with *haematoxylin* (haematoxyphilic), while protein is *acidophilic* and stains strongly with *eosin* (eosinophilic). (H & E is the customary abbreviation for the standard *haematoxylin and eosin* stain.) This mixing of red and blue colour in the cytoplasm results in purple. The plentiful cytoplasmic protein and RNA reflects the function of plasma cells as producers of large quantities of the protein *immunoglobulin* (*antibody*).

B = True   The *Golgi apparatus*, consisting mainly of flattened cisterns of lipid bilayer membrane, is generally unstained in routine sections. The 'negative image' seen in plasma cells is due partly to the large size of the Golgi apparatus and partly to the strong staining of the surrounding cytoplasm. The Golgi apparatus is important in the production of immunoglobulins. In the Golgi apparatus, covalent bonds between the *light* and *heavy immunoglobulin chains* are formed and carbohydrate side-chains are added to produce the final glycoprotein structure.

C = True   The nucleus of the plasma cell contains both *euchromatin* and *heterochromatin*. Heterochromatin refers to the dense, darkly stained areas seen around the periphery of the nucleus giving it the characteristic 'clock face' appearance. Heterochromatin represents densely coiled chromosomes and their associated proteins. Euchromatin is the name given to the paler areas of the nucleus. In these areas the chromosomes are unravelled so that a complementary RNA copy of the DNA can be produced. This *messenger RNA* (mRNA) is the template or code from which the amino acid sequence is read during protein synthesis.

D = False   This is the nucleus. All proteins are synthesised in the cytoplasm either on free *ribosomes* or on *rough endoplasmic reticulum* (*rER*).

E = False   Immunoglobulins are synthesised by rER and packaged by the Golgi apparatus (after final structural modifications) into membrane-bound vesicles. Immunoglobulins destined for release into the extracellular space are found within the lumen of the vesicles. The vesicles move to the periphery of the cell and fuse with the plasma membrane, in the process turning themselves inside out and releasing their contents into the external environment. A small proportion of immunoglobulin molecules are specifically synthesised for expression on the plasma membrane of the cell. These molecules have an extra hydrophobic section at the end of the constant region, which remains embedded in the membrane of the rER after synthesis. Once the immunoglobulin molecules are completed in the Golgi apparatus, the transport vesicle moves towards the plasma membrane. Again, when fusion with the plasma membrane takes place, the transport vesicle turns inside out and the immunoglobulins anchored in the lipid membrane are now exposed on the outer surface of the cell.

PAPER 5　　ANSWER 5.2

A = True　　This is a *neutrophil myelocyte*. It is recognisable as such by its large eccentric nucleus and prominent *azurophilic cytoplasmic granules* (see E below). The cytoplasm also contains a prominent *Golgi apparatus* identifiable as a pale area of cytoplasm adjacent to the nucleus. The Golgi apparatus consists primarily of lipid and thus does not stain with routine methods. The subsequent stages of neutrophil development are, in order, *metamyelocyte*, *stab cell* (*band form*) and *neutrophil*. The other granulocytes go through similar stages of maturation in the bone marrow and are identifiable as they mature by their different cytoplasmic granules.

B = False　　This is a *metamyelocyte*. *Osteoclasts* are found closely apposed to the margins of the bony trabeculae and are seldom seen in bone marrow aspirates. Osteoclasts are multinucleated giant cells of the monocyte–macrophage lineage.

C = False　　This cell is a myelocyte. *Haemoglobin* is only found in erythrocytes and their precursors. Haemoglobin appears in the cytoplasm at the *early normoblast* stage of erythrocyte development and increases in amount through the *late normoblast* stage. Haemoglobin production is completed during the *reticulocyte* stage. Once the nucleus has been extruded, the genes for haemoglobin are no longer available for new haemoglobin synthesis.

D = True　　**Z** identifies an *intermediate normoblast*. These cells contain increasing amounts of haemoglobin and so have *polychromatic cytoplasm*. The next stage is the *late normoblast* followed by the *reticulocyte* and then the mature erythrocyte.

E = False　　Cytoplasmic granules are characteristic of the myeloid cell series (neutrophils, eosinophils and basophils) and monocytes. No membrane bound cytoplasmic granules (lysosomes, secondary granules) are found in erythrocytes or their precursors. Reticulocytes contain a reticular precipitate that represents precipitated rRNA remnants when viewed by the supravital staining technique. However, these cells should be easily recognisable by their lack of nucleus, characteristic size and shape, and salmon pink cytoplasm.

A = True   This staining technique, the reticulin method, stains **reticulin** black. Reticulin is also known as **collagen type III**. Reticulin was originally thought to be a different type of fibre from collagen but is now recognised as a type of collagen.

B = False   These fibres are difficult to recognise in routine H & E (haematoxylin and eosin) sections, hence the need for a special technique to demonstrate them.

C = True   Reticulin forms a supporting meshwork for the epithelial cells of the liver. It is also prominent in the endocrine glands, dermis, lymph nodes, spleen and bone marrow as well as most supporting tissues. The branched nature of the fibres allows it to form a three-dimensional framework to support the cellular elements of tissue. Abnormalities of the reticulin framework occur early in certain diseases such as **cirrhosis** of the liver and **myelofibrosis** of the bone marrow. Thus, this staining method is routinely used for diagnostic purposes where such conditions are suspected.

D = False   Reticulin (or collagen type III) is a non-banded form of collagen. Type I collagen has a characteristic cross-banding pattern with a periodicity of 64 nm resulting from the staggered arrangement of the tropocollagen fibrils to form type I collagen fibres.

E = True   Typically the reticulin fibres in organs such as the spleen, lymph nodes and liver are anchored to the capsule of the organ and to septa. Thus the parenchyma of the organ is attached to the capsule, giving the tissue greater strength and cohesiveness.

A = True   Epithelial cells are of three general types. **Squamous cells** are flattened, appearing like a pavement of polygonal flagstones when viewed from above, **cuboidal cells** have a square outline when viewed in a section at right angles to the basement membrane (a horizontal section through the cell appears polygonal) and **columnar cells** are rectangular in vertical sections. Epithelial cells may be arranged as a single layer known as **simple** (e.g. simple columnar as in this example) or as multiple layers known as **stratified** (e.g. stratified squamous as in the skin). Other variants occur (e.g. pseudostratified columnar epithelium) where the epithelium is simple but appears stratified.

B = False   These are **simple tubular glands**. Glands consist of a duct and a secretory part (identical in this instance). The duct may be unbranched (a **simple gland**) or branched (a **compound gland**).

The secretory portions may either be **tubular** or **acinar**. Acinar refers to a roughly spherical secretory portion. So a gland may be simple tubular, simple acinar, compound tubular, compound acinar and so on. A further level of complexity lies in the fact that the secretory portion may also be branched giving rise to simple branched tubular and so on.

C = False   Most of the epithelial cells are **goblet cells** and contain plentiful cytoplasmic mucus, which gives the clear appearance to the cytoplasm. The presence of mucus is useful in differentiating **adenocarcinoma**, a malignant tumour arising from glandular epithelium, from other types of malignancies such as **squamous cell carcinoma** or **sarcoma**.

D = False   **Junctional complexes** form the attachment between adjacent cells and are usually found near the apices of the cells on the lateral membrane. Junctional complexes consist of a tight junction (**zonula occludens**), an adhering junction (**zonula adherens**) and a row of **desmosomes** or **spot adhering junctions**. **Hemidesmosomes** are found at the basal surface of the cell where they contribute to attachment to the basement membrane.

E = True   Neuroendocrine cells, which secrete locally acting hormones, are found scattered throughout the epithelium of the entire gastrointestinal tract.

PAPER 5   ANSWER 5.5

A = False   These cells are **myotubes**, a stage in the development of skeletal muscle fibres. The myotubes are seen here in a background of **primitive mesenchyme**. Myotubes are characterised by their multiple nuclei, which are lined up along the centre of the cell, giving a tube-like appearance.

B = True   Skeletal muscle in contrast to smooth muscle and cardiac muscle has its nuclei arranged at the periphery of the cell. The bulk of the cytoplasm is filled with a regular array of myofibrils arranged to give the characteristic cross-striated pattern. The nuclei in the mature cells are spindle shaped and somewhat flattened and compressed against the plasma membrane. These more primitive cells have rounder nuclei, which are arranged centrally.

C = False   The contractile proteins of skeletal muscle are synthesised after the formation of myotubes. This can be deduced from the fact that these cells have relatively little eosinophilic cytoplasm compared to mature skeletal muscle and cross-striations are not yet evident. However, at this stage of development, the muscle cells are producing the contractile proteins and will go on doing so throughout the rest of fetal development and childhood.

D = True   These cells, as mentioned above, are actively synthesising
            contractile proteins and therefore contain mRNA for the synthesis
            of these proteins. Protein synthesis occurs by transcription of the
            DNA to form an mRNA template. This occurs within the nucleus.
            The mRNA then migrates to the cytoplasm and intrinsic proteins
            of the cell are synthesised on free ribosomes. The mRNA cannot
            be detected in a routine H & E stained section, but its presence
            may be deduced.

E = True   The myotubes are formed by fusion of precursor cells known as
            myoblasts. These are derived from **mesenchymal cells**.
            Myoblasts are more primitive precursor cells showing less
            evidence of skeletal muscle differentiation. The myoblasts
            proliferate by mitosis and then fuse together end to end to form
            myotubes. Myoblasts have a single nucleus.

PAPER 5	ANSWER 5.6

A = False   This micrograph shows a **peripheral ganglion** at high power. The
            cells marked **X** are **satellite cells**, which serve to provide
            metabolic and structural support to the ganglion cells.
            Oligodendrocytes are found in the central nervous system and
            perform a similar function to the **Schwann cells** of peripheral
            nerve tissue, i.e. the formation of myelin sheaths and insulation of
            non-myelinated nerve fibres by enclosing the nerve fibres within
            their cytoplasm.

B = False   The **substantia nigra**, part of the midbrain of the central
            nervous system, contains pigmented nerve cells. Obviously this
            cannot be substantia nigra as the micrograph is identified as
            being peripheral nerve tissue. The cells pictured here are
            ganglion cells from a **sympathetic ganglion**. Pigment is not
            found in parasympathetic ganglion cells nor in somatic sensory
            ganglia.

C = True   The cell bodies of ganglion cells (nerve cells), as seen here, are
            round with large slightly eccentric nuclei with very large nucleoli.
            This enables nerve cells to be easily identified in tissue sections
            even when present as very small aggregates (as between the
            two layers of the muscularis propria in the gastrointestinal tract)
            or as single cells (as in the submucosa of the gastrointestinal
            tract).

D = False   The brown pigment is **lipofuscin**. Lipofuscin is a 'wear and tear'
            pigment found in the cytoplasm of ganglion cells of sympathetic
            ganglia of the autonomic nervous system. Parasympathetic
            ganglion cells do not contain obvious lipofuscin. The highly
            pigmented nerve cells in the substantia nigra of the midbrain
            contain neuromelanin pigment rather than lipofuscin.

E = True   The loose collagenous supporting tissue between the ganglion cells contains an extensive network of *axons* and *dendrites*. The axons include the axons of nerve fibres entering and leaving the ganglion, which synapse with the ganglion cells. The dendrites form synapses with other ganglion cells.

PAPER 5	ANSWER 5.7

A = True   This is an *elastic artery*. The aorta, innominate, common carotid and subclavian arteries are all elastic arteries. The *tunica media* of these vessels is arranged in concentric sheets of elastin, which is responsible for elastic recoil of the arteries thus maintaining the systemic blood pressure during diastole. The *tunicae intima* and *adventitia* have the same structure as other arteries.

B = False   The radial artery, along with the femoral, coronary and cerebral arteries, is a *muscular artery*. In muscular arteries, the elastic tissue is arranged as two distinct layers: the *internal elastic lamina* separating the tunica intima from the tunica media and the *external elastic lamina* between the tunicae media and adventitia. The bulk of the tunica media in muscular arteries consists, not surprisingly, of smooth muscle which, under the control of the sympathetic nervous system and adrenal medullary hormones, controls the flow of blood to the organs.

C = True   The intima is similar in all arteries. There is a layer of flattened endothelial cells resting on a thin layer of supporting tissue rich in elastin. At this magnification the endothelial cells cannot really be distinguished. This supporting tissue contains occasional fibroblasts as well as cells known as *myointimal cells*, which have features on electron microscopy similar to smooth muscle cells.

D = True   The adventitia of elastic arteries contains *vasa vasorum*, small arteries which run in the adventitia and outer tunica media, supplying them with oxygen and nutrients. An example can just be seen at the lower right corner of the micrograph. The wall of the elastic arteries is too thick for supply of oxygen and nutrients from the blood in the lumen of the artery. Thus the inner half of the tunica media is supplied by luminal blood and the outer half by the vasa vasorum. The tunica adventitia also contains collagen and elastin and merges imperceptibly with surrounding supporting tissue.

E = False   The tunica media of elastic arteries consists of layers of smooth muscle and collagen between the concentric sheets of elastin. Although there is generally less smooth muscle in these vessels than in the muscular arteries, the smooth muscle is still a substantial component of the media. Transition from elastic to muscular arteries is a gradual process and in general as the amount of elastin in the vessel wall decreases, the amount of smooth muscle becomes relatively greater.

PAPER 5   ANSWER 5.8

A = False   This is the ***papillary dermis***. The ***reticular dermis*** is the thicker deep part of the dermis that provides most of the mechanical support for the skin. The reticular dermis consists of coarse bundles of collagen. The papillary dermis is the thin superficial layer of the dermis immediately deep to the epidermis and is composed of more delicate collagen bundles than the reticular dermis.

B = False   This is a ***sebaceous gland***. These are usually closely associated with hair follicles and can be identified by the characteristic pale cytoplasm of the secretory cells. A hair follicle cut in oblique section can be seen adjacent to this sebaceous gland. Sebaceous glands usually empty their secretions (***sebum***) into the hair follicle. Sebum is an oily substance that has a waterproofing function on the skin. The secretory epithelial cells have cytoplasm packed with lipid vacuoles that give the cells their pale foamy cytoplasm. The lipid material is secreted by disintegration of the cell (***holocrine secretion***).

C = True   The epidermis and papillary dermis have an undulating interface. ***Dermal papillae*** arising from the papillary dermis interdigitate with ***rete ridges*** extending downwards from the epidermis. This arrangement increases the tensile strength of the skin. The dermal papillae contain capillary loops, which arise from the papillary vascular plexus and lie very close to the basement membrane of the epidermis, thus improving the transfer of nutrients and metabolic products to and from the epidermis.

D = False   There are two major vascular plexuses in the skin. The ***papillary (subpapillary) plexus*** is found in the upper part of the dermis, approximately at the junction of the reticular and papillary dermis. This plexus of small vessels gives rise to the capillaries of the dermal papillae. The ***cutaneous plexus***, composed of larger vessels, is found at the interface of the dermis and ***subcutis (hypodermis)***.

E = False   **W** marks an ***eccrine (merocrine) sweat gland***. These are coiled tubular glands which lie in the subcutis and secrete a watery fluid (sweat). Active transport of sodium ions by the secretory cells into the gland lumen leads to passive diffusion of water. The sweat is then modified by reabsorption of sodium ions in the excretory ducts, which are impermeable to water. Decapitation or ***apocrine secretion*** is characteristic of ***apocrine sweat glands***.

222

A = True   The **germinal centre** is found in activated or **secondary lymphoid follicles** and contains activated B lymphocytes. These B lymphocytes are dividing and maturing in response to one or more antigens. The end result is the production of clones of **memory cells** and **plasma cells**, which are able to produce large amounts of antibody. The activated cells in the germinal centre are larger and less closely packed than the surrounding inactive B cells and therefore appear a paler shade of brown.

B = False   This is the **interfollicular zone**, which is part of the **paracortex**. This area is the domain of T lymphocytes, which do not bind to the specific anti-B cell antibody used in this preparation and therefore are not stained brown. T lymphocytes do not form follicles but in response to certain antigens (e.g. viral infection, delayed hypersensitivity reactions) the paracortex may become expanded by activated T lymphocytes which divide and mature to produce effector T lymphocytes such as **cytotoxic T cells** or **helper T cells**.

C = False   Although the germinal centre contains large numbers of B lymphocytes, several other cell types are also found here and are necessary for B lymphocyte activation and division. These include T helper cells, **follicular dendritic cells**, which present antigen on their surface to lymphocytes, and **tingible body macrophages**, which phagocytose cellular debris generated by apoptotic cells.

D = False   **Z** marks the **mantle zone** of the follicle, which immediately surrounds the germinal centre. The mantle zone consists of small inactive B lymphocytes. The **marginal zone** of a lymphoid follicle is peripheral to the mantle zone and is very ill defined in lymph node follicles. However, in the spleen the marginal zone is well defined.

E = True   **High endothelial venules** (**HEV**) are found in the interfollicular or paracortical area of the lymph node. This area is primarily populated by T lymphocytes. HEV, not easily identified in this type of preparation, are small **postcapillary venules** lined by cuboidal rather than squamous endothelium. HEV are a major site of lymphocyte entry into the lymph node. The cuboidal epithelium expresses surface receptors for lymphocyte, cutely known as '**addressins**'. Lymphocytes bearing the appropriate addressins bind to the endothelial receptors and are triggered to pass through the wall of the HEV into the lymph node. The addressin system is the main mechanism whereby lymphocyte trafficking is regulated.

A = True   The **pulmonary arteries** are wide-calibre arteries with approximately the same diameter as the bronchus or bronchiole they accompany. Hence the pulmonary blood pressure is much lower than systemic blood pressure. Two slightly oblique cross-sections of this pulmonary artery branch are seen in this micrograph. The oblique nature of the section makes the artery appear larger than the bronchiole it accompanies. The blood within the arteries is stained yellow by this method.

B = False   This is a **bronchiole**. **Bronchi** have hyaline cartilage in their wall, which helps to prevent collapse of the bronchus during expiration. Bronchioles are of smaller calibre with no cartilage. The elastic tissue of the lung helps to hold the bronchioles patent during expiration.

C = False   This structure is an **alveolus**, which in life is filled with air. Blood circulates in the huge network of tiny capillaries found within the alveolar walls (not seen at this magnification). Only a very thin layer of tissue separates the air from the capillary blood, facilitating diffusion of gases between the air and the blood.

D = True   The air side of the alveolar wall has an epithelial lining of **type I pneumocytes**. These squamous epithelial cells and their basement membranes form part of the alveolar wall. Between the two layers of epithelium and basement membrane lie the alveolar capillaries and a small amount of supporting tissue. **Type II pneumocytes** are also found in small numbers. These rounded calls produce **surfactant**, which lowers surface tension in the alveolus helping to prevent collapse of the alveolus in expiration.

E = True   Pulmonary arteries are classified as **elastic arteries**. Compared to a systemic artery of the same calibre, they have less smooth muscle and more elastin in their walls. Thus their wall structure most nearly resembles elastic arteries, such as the aorta, rather than **muscular arteries** like the femoral artery.

PAPER 5   ANSWER 5.11

A = False   This is a **circumvallate papilla**. The **filiform papillae** have a pointed structure surmounted by a steeple-like arrangement of keratin. **Fungiform papillae** have a globular shape. Fungiform and filiform papillae are plentiful in the anterior two-thirds of the tongue and are not seen in this micrograph. Circumvallate papillae contain most of the taste buds in the tongue.

B = True   Large numbers of specialised nerve cells (**gustatory cells**) and their supporting cells (**sustentacular cells**) are found in the stratified squamous epithelium of the sides of the circumvallate papillae. These cells are gathered together into groups of about 50 cells to form the barrel-shaped taste buds. The nerve cells are specialised **chemoreceptors**. Food dissolved in saliva enters the taste bud through the taste pore at the surface and stimulates the sensory nerve cells. Taste buds are found in other parts of the tongue and other areas of the mouth but the main concentration is found in the epithelium of the circumvallate papillae.

C = False   The circumvallate papillae are found in a row immediately anterior to the **sulcus terminalis**, a V-shaped groove that defines the border between the anterior two-thirds and the posterior one-third of the tongue. The mucosa of the anterior two-thirds of the tongue contains large numbers of filiform and fungiform papillae.

D = False   The tongue, like most of the oral cavity, is lined by a **stratified squamous epithelium** supported by a collagenous lamina propria, which together make up the oral mucosa. The inherent toughness of stratified squamous epithelium is required in this area to withstand the friction on the epithelium during mastication. In some species with a particularly coarse diet, e.g. rodents, the oral mucosa is keratinised.

E = False   Food substances dissolve in the watery fluid secreted by the **serous salivary glands** lying under the mucosa. The glands around the circumvallate papillae are called **von Ebner's glands** and empty into the cleft around the papilla via a duct, which is easily seen in this micrograph. Mucous glands, which are not seen in this micrograph, can be easily recognised by their clear, somewhat granular cytoplasm.

PAPER 5	ANSWER 5.12

A = False   **Enterocytes** are the main absorptive cells in the small intestine, and are tall columnar cells with a prominent brush border of surface microvilli. In contrast, the epithelial cells of the colon are a mixture of **goblet cells**, which produce mucin, and **absorptive cells**. Both of these cell types are tall columnar in form. Goblet cells are easily recognised by their supranuclear goblet-shaped collection of mucus. Both the absorptive and the goblet cells have small numbers of surface microvilli but these are present in insufficient numbers to form a brush border visible by light microscopy.

B = True   The normal population of cells in the **lamina propria** includes plasma cells along with lymphocytes and small numbers of eosinophils. These cells, along with organised lymphoid aggregates, contribute to the immune defence system of the colon. The plasma cells secrete immunoglobulins, mainly of **secretory IgA** class, into the lumen of the bowel as well as into the blood. The lymphoid aggregates are smaller than the **Peyer's patches** of the small intestine.

C = False   The **muscularis propria** is not seen in this micrograph. The fine layer of smooth muscle marked **X** is the **muscularis mucosae**, which along with the epithelium and lamina propria, makes up the

mucosa of the colon. The muscularis propria is separated from the muscularis mucosa by the **submucosa**, consisting of loose connective tissue containing larger blood vessels and nerve fibres. In the colon as in the rest of the gastrointestinal tract, the muscularis propria consists of an **inner circular layer** and an **outer longitudinal layer**. A feature unique to the colon is that the outer longitudinal layer is divided into three longitudinal bands of muscle known as **teniae coli**.

D = False   The crypts are in the form of straight tubular glands in the normal colon, although branching may occur in some disease states, such as the chronic inflammatory condition, **ulcerative colitis**.

E = True   The intestinal contents are progressively dehydrated as they pass through the colon, from liquid at the **ileocaecal valve**, to solid at the rectum. Thus one major function of the absorptive cells is to remove water from the lumen of the colon. To facilitate this, the surface cells are mainly absorptive cells, whereas the goblet cells are predominant in the lining of the crypts.

PAPER 5   ANSWER 5.13

A = True   This cell is a **parietal cell**, which is easily recognisable in an H & E stained section by its 'fried egg' appearance. It is characterised by extensive eosinophilic cytoplasm and a central round nucleus. These cells are found in the stomach, mainly in the body and fundus but small numbers may be seen in gastric antral mucosa. The cytoplasm contains deep branching canaliculi, which form a network throughout the cytoplasm and are in continuity with the lumen of the gland. The **canalicular system** together with the associated **tubulovesicular membrane complex** is the acid-secreting mechanism of the stomach.

B = False   This is a **peptic (chief, zymogenic)** cell recognisable by its basophilic cytoplasm and basal nucleus. These cells are found in the base of the glands in the gastric body and fundus. These cells secrete the proenzyme **pepsinogen**, which in the acid environment of the stomach is converted to **pepsin**. **Intrinsic factor** is a product of parietal cells. Intrinsic factor binds to vitamin B_{12} in the stomach and is necessary for absorption of B_{12} in the terminal ileum.

C = False   **Gastrin** is secreted by neuroendocrine cells in the gastric antrum. These cells are found scattered between the bases of the other epithelial cells and secrete gastrin in response to the presence of food in the stomach. Gastrin acts on both parietal and peptic cells in the body of the stomach to increase their secretions.

D = False   Mucin secretion in the gastric body is a function of **surface mucous** and **neck mucous cells**. As one would expect, these tall columnar cells have pale cytoplasm because of the mucus content (but are not goblet cells). The nucleus is in the base of the cell. Surface and neck mucous cells appear similar by light microscopy but neck mucous cells have larger secretory granules and more polyribosomes when examined by electron microscopy.

E = False   Parietal cells do not divide. The **reserve** or **stem cells** of the gastric glands are found in the neck of the glands. These small inconspicuous epithelial cells divide continuously to replace dead cells in the rest of the epithelium. The cells so produced may migrate towards the surface or base of the gland and differentiate into any of the other cell types found there.

PAPER 5   ANSWER 5.14

A = True   The bulk of the **lens** of the eye is composed of lens fibres packed with **crystallins**. The fibres are elongated prisms that have developed from the posterior cells of the lens. As the lens develops, these cells elongate so as to lie with their long axis in the anteroposterior axis. The cell nuclei are lost and the plasma membranes of the cells fuse leaving a mass of optically clear crystals with very little interstitial substance.

B = True   The lens is attached to the **ciliary body** by the **suspensory ligament**. The ciliary body is a ring of smooth muscle around the coronal equator of the lens. Contraction and relaxation of this muscle alters the shape of the lens so as to focus the incident light on the retina.

C = True   The lens is encased in a thick basement membrane known as the **lens capsule**.

D = False   This is the **anterior cuboidal epithelium**. There is no epithelial cell layer on the posterior surface of the adult lens. The posterior cells of the lens lose their nuclei as mentioned above and become the substrate of the lens.

E = False   The lens forms in the early embryo from a single layer of epithelium derived from **ectoderm**. The cells destined to become the lens form an invagination in the ectoderm, known as the **lens pit**. This breaks free forming the **lens vesicle** and sinks into the **optic vesicle**. The posterior cells then begin their development into lens fibres as described above.

PAPER 5   ANSWER 5.15

A = True   This is a **collecting duct**. Collecting ducts are lined by a tall columnar epithelium with pale-staining cytoplasm. **Collecting**

tubules, which drain into collecting ducts, have a cuboidal epithelium indistinguishable from the epithelium of the **thick ascending limb of the loop of Henle**. The collecting tubule, however, can be distinguished from the thick ascending limb by its wider diameter and less regular shape.

B = True   The **thin limbs of the loop of Henle** are small-diameter tubules lined by flattened squamous epithelium. They are indistinguishable from the **vasa recta** except that vasa recta contain erythrocytes. Several vasa recta filled with blood can be identified in this micrograph as bright carmine-stained areas.

C = True   The collecting tubules and collecting ducts are both responsive to **antidiuretic hormone** (**ADH** or **vasopressin**). It is in this segment of the renal tubule that the final concentration of the urine is determined. In the presence of ADH, the epithelium of the collecting tubule and the proximal part of the duct becomes more permeable to water, and water thus passively diffuses into the hyperosmolar medullary interstitium. If the body is dehydrated, ADH is secreted and water is retained by the body. In a situation of relative overhydration, ADH is not secreted and a more dilute urine is passed, expelling excess water from the body.

D = True   The interstitium of the medulla, stained blue by this method, contains a high concentration of urea relative to the thin limbs of the loop of Henle. In the presence of ADH, the collecting tubules and ducts are permeable to water, which is drawn passively into the interstitium by the hyperosmolar medullary interstitium. This water is returned to the circulation by the vasa recta. The urea in the interstitium diffuses passively from the collecting duct along its concentration gradient, as the concentration of urea is even higher in the collecting duct.

E = False   This is one of the thin limbs of the loop of Henle. The epithelium is simple squamous in type and these cells do not actively transport sodium ions from the urine. Ultrastructurally this lack of active transport is reflected in the scanty mitochondria and lack of the basolateral interdigitations that are seen in other parts of the renal tubule (the thick ascending limb, the distal convoluted tubule, the collecting tubule and the proximal convoluted tubule). The epithelium of the thin descending limb is permeable to water, allowing passive diffusion of water into the interstitium, while the shorter thin ascending limb is not permeable to water.

A = True   These calcified structures, known as **pineal sand**, accumulate in the pineal gland with age. They consist of an organic matrix containing calcium and magnesium phosphate. This histological appearance of calcification is also typical of calcification in pathological conditions (e.g. in breast carcinoma or dystrophic calcification in blood vessels) and can be recognised by the strong staining of the structure and the very well defined edge. The calcification of the pineal is useful in adults to determine on skull X-rays if there has been swelling of one half of the brain, which pushes the pineal (made visible by calcification) to the other side.

B = True   These cells, which form clusters in the pineal, are known as *pinealocytes* or *pineal chief cells*. These cells secrete the hormone *melatonin*.

C = True   The pinealocytes are responsive to light and dark, secreting melatonin at night but not in the daytime. Melatonin causes drowsiness and sleep and thus controls the *circadian rhythm* of the body. Thus the pineal acts as a neuroendocrine transducer, converting a neurological signal, triggered by light falling on the retina, into a chemical signal (the hormone melatonin).

D = False   These cells are *neuroglial cells* similar to *astrocytes* in the rest of the central nervous system. The pinealocytes are very specialised nerve cells and are supported by the neuroglial cells as astrocytes support neurones of the central nervous system.

E = True   The hormone melatonin, secreted by pinealocytes, has other functions in addition to regulation of circadian rhythm. Melatonin in some reptiles and lower vertebrates controls skin colour by regulation of the synthesis of melanin. Other functions include regulation of the reproductive cycle of animals which reproduce seasonally and regulation of ageing, the immune system and puberty in humans.

PAPER 5	ANSWER 5.17

A = True   This is a *seminiferous tubule* where male gametes are produced. Undifferentiated germ cells line the tubule and divide continuously after puberty to produce *spermatozoa*. Various cell types are identifiable (although not at this power) in the production of spermatozoa. The most primitive cells, *type A spermatogonia*, divide to produce more type A spermatogonia as well as more differentiated *type B spermatogonia*. These undergo further cycles of mitotic division to produce *primary spermatocytes*. Primary spermatocytes undergo the first meiotic division, giving rise to *secondary spermatocytes* that immediately undergo a second meiotic division to produce *spermatids*, which finally mature into spermatozoa.

B = False   *Leydig cells* are found in the interstitium of the testis **Y**, between the seminiferous tubules (see E below). *Sertoli cells* are the other major cell type (besides germ cells) found within the seminiferous tubule. Sertoli cells perform multiple functions necessary for the production of spermatozoa, including secretion of regulatory factors. Sertoli cells also regulate Leydig cell function, produce **inhibin**, secrete tubular fluid, and divide the lining of the seminiferous tubule into two compartments, the **basal** and **adluminal compartments**.

C = False   Each primary spermatocyte produces four haploid gametes, **spermatozoa**, during the two meiotic divisions. This is not surprising considering the large numbers of spermatozoa produced daily by a normal adult human male. In women, however, much smaller numbers of germ cells are produced and each **ovum** requires a large amount of cytoplasm for nutritional support until implantation has occurred. Thus in females two meiotic divisions give rise to one ovum and three **polar bodies**.

D = False   The wall of the seminiferous tubule consists of a basement membrane surrounded by fibroblasts and myofibroblasts, which do contribute some contractile function. However, there are no distinct layers of smooth muscle.

E = True   Leydig cells are found in the interstitium of the testis occurring as single cells or small groups. These cells secrete the male sex hormone testosterone and are responsive to **luteinising hormone** (**LH**) secreted by the pituitary. In males LH is sometimes known as **interstitial cell stimulating hormone** (**ICSH**). Leydig cells have the typical ultrastructure of steroid-secreting cells with plentiful cytoplasmic smooth endoplasmic reticulum. Another unique factor of these cells, found only in humans and wild bush rats, is the presence of **crystals of Reinke** in the cytoplasm. These can be seen with light microscopy when suitable stains are used.

PAPER 5	ANSWER 5.18

A = False   This structure is a **corpus albicans**, which results from the regression of a **corpus luteum**. The corpus albicans consists of pale inactive fibrous tissue containing very few cells. By contrast, the corpus luteum is a cellular structure consisting of **luteinised granulosa** and **theca interna cells**, which produce progesterone and oestrogen respectively.

B = False   These stromal cells of the ovary are quite different from endometrial stromal cells. Morphologically they are spindle-shaped cells, some of which contain cytoplasmic lipid, as opposed to the oval shape of the endometrial stroma. More importantly, ovarian stromal cells adjacent to a developing follicle differentiate into theca cells, which produce the hormones oestrogen and oestrogen precursors, some progesterone, FSH and inhibin F at different points in the menstrual cycle.

C = True   As mentioned above, ovarian stromal cells are part of a major endocrine organ producing different hormones, including oestrogen and progesterone at different stages of the menstrual cycle. During their active secretory phase they develop the ultrastructural features of typical steroid-secreting cells, i.e. plentiful intracellular lipid and smooth endoplasmic reticulum (sER), a morphological appearance known as **luteinisation** (only applied to ovarian granulosa and theca cells and not to other steroid-hormone-secreting cells).

D = False   Although many corpora albicantes (plural of corpus albicans) may be found in the ovaries of elderly women, a large proportion of them atrophy and disappear completely. If they all persisted the average postmenopausal woman would have approximately 500 corpora albicantes.

E = False   Ova are produced by germ cells (**primary oocytes**) found in primordial follicles in the outer cortex of the ovary (not included in this micrograph). The primordial follicle consists of the primary oocyte and a surrounding layer of **follicular cells**. In women of reproductive age, a number of primary oocytes begin maturing into ova with each menstrual cycle. The surrounding follicular cells and adjacent theca cells also differentiate and form the corpus luteum after the ovum has been ejected into the peritoneal cavity. Although about 20 oocytes begin maturation in each cycle usually only one reaches maturity, with the rest degenerating (**atretic follicles**).

PAPER 5   ANSWER 5.19

A = True   The **granular layer** of the cerebellum is very cellular, the closely packed cell nuclei giving it a deep blue colour in this routine H & E stained slide. The cells comprising the granular layer are small neurones. Afferent nerve axons reach the cerebellum and synapse with these small neurones in the cerebellum, each axon synapsing with more than one granular layer neurone.

B = False   The area marked **Y** is the **molecular layer** and contains scanty neurones including specialised types known as **stellate cells** and **basket cells**. The bulk of the tissue of the molecular layer consists of non-myelinated axons of the granular cell neurones and dendrites of the **Purkinje cells**. These axons and dendrites, as well as the processes of the stellate and basket cells, form multiple synapses with each other in order to integrate incoming signals relating to posture and motion and generate outgoing signals, which control balance and posture as well as muscular activity.

C = True   Purkinje cells are very large neurones, the cell bodies of which
           are found at the junction of the granular and molecular layers of
           the cerebellar cortex. The numerous dendrites of the Purkinje
           cells pass into the molecular layer and participate in the complex
           network of synapses found there. Each Purkinje cell has a single
           fine axon that passes through the granular cell layer into the
           white matter of the *cerebellar medulla*. The axons of the
           Purkinje cells are the only efferent nerve fibres from the
           cerebellum. They pass to the central nuclei of the cerebellum
           where they synapse.

D = False   The tissue marked **Z** is the medulla of the cerebellum. Although it
           contains many unmyelinated nerve fibres, the majority are
           myelinated, giving it its white appearance macroscopically in a
           similar fashion to the white matter of the cerebral medulla.

E = False   *Golgi cells* are one of the types of neurones found in the
           superficial part of the granular layer of the cerebellum.

PAPER 5   ANSWER 5.20

A = False   The area marked **X** is the *zona fasciculata*. The cells in this layer
           are arranged in long columns. Between the columns of steroid-
           hormone-secreting epithelial cells, there is a network of wide
           capillaries (sinusoids) which enable the rapid secretion of the
           hormones into the blood. The sinusoids arise from the
           subcapsular vascular plexus and run through the cortex
           towards the medulla where they drain eventually into the *central
           vein of the medulla*.

B = False   This is the *zona glomerulosa*, the most superficial layer of the
           adrenal cortex. The cells in this layer are responsible for the
           secretion of *aldosterone* (see C below). In this layer, which is
           often incomplete, the secretory cells are arranged in small ovoid
           clusters.

C = False   The zona glomerulosa, the outermost layer of the cortex,
           secretes aldosterone. Aldosterone is important in the control of
           blood pressure and forms part of the renin–angiotensin–
           aldosterone mechanism. *Adrenaline* (and *noradrenaline*) are
           products of the *adrenal medulla*, which is not included in this
           micrograph. The cells of the adrenal medulla are in intimate
           contact with preganglionic sympathetic nerve fibres. Nerve
           impulses initiate release of adrenaline and noradrenaline, giving
           rise to the familiar 'fight or flight reaction'.

D = True   The endocrine cells of the adrenal cortex, including the zona
           fasciculata, are steroid-hormone-secreting cells. These cells
           contain plentiful smooth endoplasmic reticulum, the site of
           synthesis of steroid hormones. These cells of the zona fasciculata

also contain plentiful lipid droplets in their cytoplasm. Thus the cells of the zona fasciculata have paler cytoplasm than cells in the other layers of the cortex.

E = True   The adrenal gland is supplied by branches of the **superior**, **middle** and **inferior suprarenal arteries**. These give rise to **long** and **short cortical arteries**. The short cortical arteries feed into the subcapsular plexus, which in turn supplies the capillaries (sinusoids) that ramify through the cortex, draining eventually into the central vein of the medulla. The long cortical arteries traverse the cortex and supply the capillaries in the medulla. Again, the drainage from these vessels is into the central vein of the medulla.

PAPER 5   ANSWER 5.21

A = True   The micrograph shows the surface of **enterocytes** of the small bowel. The surface has large numbers of **microvilli**, which are shown here in slightly oblique section. Nevertheless, the elongated structure of the microvilli can be appreciated and it is easy to see the central core of **actin microfilaments**. The **terminal web** is also well demonstrated in the upper cytoplasm.

B = False   This is a **desmosome** (**macula adherens**), which is the third part of the **junctional complex** found between adjacent epithelial cells near the lumen of the small bowel, as well as in many other types of epithelia. Desmosomes in this area are arranged in a circle around the upper part of the cell, joining it to all the cells with which it comes in contact. Desmosomes are also found scattered at random along the lateral plasma membrane of the cell where they perform the same function. The desmosome is connected to the **intermediate filaments** of the **cytoskeleton** on the cytoplasmic side and to the adjacent cell by fine filaments called **transmembrane linkers**.

C = False   This is an **occluding junction** (**tight junction, zonula occludens**) which forms the first part of the junctional complex. The major function of the occluding junction is, as its name suggests, to seal the intercellular space so that the contents of the lumen of the bowel cannot enter the lateral space between adjacent cells. In occluding junctions, the plasma membranes of the two cells are very close together and appear sometimes to fuse. This is due to the presence of fine ridges in the membranes. Known as **sealing strands**, these ridges represent a complementary pair of membrane proteins tightly linked together.

D = True   **Hemidesmosomes** are found at the base of the cell and link it to the basement membrane. As their name suggests, these structures are half a desmosome. Like desmosomes they are connected to the intermediate filaments of the cytoskeleton. They bind to the *lamina densa* of the basement membrane by means of proteins called *integrins*. The basement membrane is thickened in this area.

E = True   This is a *zonula adherens* or *adhering junction* and forms the second or middle component of the junctional complex. Adhering junctions form a continuous ring around the cell and, along with desmosomes, they anchor adjacent cells to each other. As with desmosomes there is slight separation of the plasma membranes of the two cells. This space is filled by an unknown substance that binds the two cells together. On the cytoplasmic side the adhering junction is connected to the cytoskeleton of the cell. The combination of adhering junctions and desmosomes provides the tensile strength to form a highly cohesive epithelium.

PAPER 5   ANSWER 5.22

A = True   The outer membrane of mitochondria is more permeable than the inner membrane. The permeability is due to pores in the outer membrane that are formed by the protein *porin*. These pores allow free passage of small molecules through the outer membrane. The inner membrane of the mitochondrion is folded into *cristae*, which can be seen in this micrograph as folds of lipid membrane. The space between the inner and outer membranes is known as the *intermembranous space* and this extends into the cristae of the mitochondrion. The shape of the cristae varies in different tissues and is often characteristic of a particular cell type.

B = True   **X** is a *matrix granule*. These are found scattered throughout mitochondria and are thought to be the binding sites for calcium. Mitochondria are a major storage site for calcium ions within cells. The matrix granules are found in the *matrix* within the inner membrane.

C = True   The mitochondria are the main site of *aerobic respiration* within the cell. Aerobic respiration, carried out by the enzymes of *Krebs' cycle*, takes place mainly in the matrix of mitochondria. The enzymes of Krebs' cycle are found within the matrix along with the enzymes involved in the oxidation of fatty acids. Many of these enzymes are synthesised within the mitochondrion itself, while others are imported from the cell cytoplasm.

D = False   The small dark granules surrounding the mitochondria are *glycogen granules*. It can sometimes be difficult to discriminate between free ribosomes and glycogen granules. The presence of glycogen rosettes is often helpful. Glycogen rosettes are clusters of glycogen particles. Ribosomes are slightly larger than glycogen granules.

E = True   Mitochondria contain one or more lengths of DNA. In contrast to the DNA in the cell nucleus, the DNA in the mitochondrion is arranged in a circle, in a similar fashion to the chromosomes of bacteria. Mitochondria use this DNA to synthesise many of their enzymes. Mitochondria divide in a manner analogous to bacteria with reduplication of their DNA.

PAPER 5	ANSWER 5.23

A = True   **X** marks the ***myelin sheath***. The myelin sheath is formed from multiple layers of ***Schwann cell*** cytoplasm and plasma membrane wrapped tightly around the axon. The cytoplasm of the Schwann cell is excluded from the myelin sheath and the inner leaflets of the plasma membrane fuse together. The darker lines in the myelin sheath are termed the ***major dense lines***, and represent the fused inner leaflets of the plasma membrane. The intervening paler lines are the ***intraperiod lines*** and these represent the outer layers of the plasma membrane, which are closely apposed to each other. The myelin sheath acts as a layer of insulation around the nerve axon and is interrupted by the ***nodes of Ranvier***. Conduction of impulses along the nerve is by ***saltatory conduction*** whereby the action potential leaps from one node of Ranvier to the next. This gives rise to greatly increased velocity of nerve impulse conduction.

B = True   **Y** is the axon of a ***non-myelinated nerve*** surrounded by a thin rim of Schwann cell cytoplasm. The plasma membranes of both axon and Schwann cell can easily be identified in this micrograph. It is common to find several axons embedded within a single Schwann cell in non-myelinated nerves. You will note that myelinated and non-myelinated nerves are found close together in a single nerve bundle. This is usually the case.

C = True   **Z** marks the cytoplasm of the Schwann cell, forming the myelin sheath around the myelinated nerve fibre. In a favourable plane of section, the nucleus of the Schwann cell might be seen in the same position. Each myelinated nerve axon is surrounded by the cytoplasm of multiple Schwann cells. A single Schwann cell gives rise to the myelin sheath between two nodes of Ranvier. The node of Ranvier thus marks the junction of myelin sheath derived from two different Schwann cells.

D = True   Axons contain ***microtubules***, which are seen in both myelinated and non-myelinated fibres in this micrograph. Microtubules are easily recognised in cross-section as small hollow rounded structures. In longitudinal section, microtubules are long and non-branching and again in a favourable plane of section, can be seen to be hollow.

E = False   The structure marked **W** is a *mitochondrion*. Mitochondria are seen throughout the length of nerve axons and fulfil their usual role of providing energy. The nucleus of the axon would be found either within a peripheral ganglion or within the central nervous system.

A = True   The structures marked **X** are *chylomicrons* in the *intercellular clefts*. These are composed of triglycerides with a limiting coat of phospholipids and proteins, and are on their way to the small lymphatics just deep to the epithelium in the lamina propria of the mucosa. Chylomicrons are the main mechanism for absorption of lipids from the gut lumen.

B = True   These are *dense core granules*, which are characteristic of *neuroendocrine cells*. The central cell in this electron micrograph is therefore identified as a neuroendocrine cell, whilst the two adjacent cells, which have no dense core bodies, are *enterocytes*. As can be seen in this high-magnification micrograph, dense core granules have an electron-dense core surrounded by an electron-lucent zone with an outer lipid membrane. The dense core represents the stored secretory products of the cell, which in this case could be secretin, somatostatin, enteroglucagon or serotonin. The dense core granules are usually found at the base of the cells. Note that a small part of the nucleus of the cell can be seen at the top of the micrograph.

C = False   Neuroendocrine cells do not have the large numbers of *microvilli* that are found at the surface of enterocytes. Many of these cells do not actually reach the lumen of the bowel (*closed-type neuroendocrine cells*). Others do extend to the surface and may be responsive to the contents of the gut (*open-type neuroendocrine cells*).

D = False   Chylomicrons are assembled within the enterocytes from lipid absorbed from the gut lumen. *Triglycerides* in the gut lumen are broken down into a monoglyceride plus two free fatty acids by lipases secreted by the pancreas. The lipids are absorbed into the enterocytes, resynthesised into triglycerides and formed into chylomicrons. The triglycerides pass into the intercellular cleft and through the basement membrane to reach small lacteals in the lamina propria. In this micrograph, chylomicrons can be seen 'queuing' up on the epithelial side of the basement membrane to pass through it.

E = True   **Z** is the *lamina densa* of the epithelial basement membrane and is separated from the epithelium by the *lamina lucida*. The third layer is the *lamina fibroreticularis*, which merges into the underlying supporting tissue and can barely be resolved at this magnification.

INDEX

Mitosis, 2.3, 3.16, 4.1, 4.3
Mitotic spindle, 4.1
Monocytes, 4.2
Motor (efferent) nerve fibres, 4.5
Mucociliary escalator, 1.11, 2.4
Mucosa-associated lymphoid tissue (MALT), 1.1, 3.9
Mucus secretion, 2.4, 4.11, 5.13
Muller cells, 4.19
Muscular arteries, 4.6, 5.7, 5.10
Muscularis mucosa, 5.12
Muscularis propria, 1.14, 3.11, 4.12, 5.12
Myelin sheath, 2.24, 4.5, 5.23
Myelinated nerve fibres, 4.5
Myelocytes, 5.2
Myelofibrosis, 5.3
Myenteric (Auerbach's) plexus, 1.14, 3.11
Myoblasts, 5.5
Myocardium, 1.8
Myoepithelial cells, 4.18
    dilator pupillae, 1.19
    salivary glands, 1.12
Myofibrils, 1.22, 1.23
    cardiac muscle, 2.5
Myointimal cells, 5.7
Myometrium, 4.4, 4.20
Myosin, 3.20, 5.5
    mesangial cells, 3.24
    skeletal muscle, 1.22
    smooth muscle, 2.21
Myotubes, 5.5

Necrosis, 2.3
Negative selection/clonal deletion, 1.10
Neuroendocrine cells, 1.16, 4.13
    dense core granules, 3.10, 5.24
    gastrointestinal epithelium, 1.14, 2.12, 3.11, 4.11, 5.4, 5.24
    respiratory epithelium, 1.11, 2.4
Neurofilament proteins, 2.24
Neuroglial cells, 5.16
Neuromuscular junction, 1.23
Neurone, 1.18, 3.5
Neuropil, 1.18, 3.5
Neurotransmission, 1.18
Neutrophil myelocyte, 5.2
Neutrophils, 1.2, 2.22
    maturation, 5.2
Nexus (gap) junctions, 2.21, 3.21
Nissl bodies, 3.5
Nitrous oxide, 4.24
Nodes of Ranvier, 5.23
Non-histone proteins, 4.23

Non-myelinated nerve, 4.5, 5.23
Noradrenaline (norepinephrine), 2.15, 5.20
Normoblast, 5.2
Nuclear membrane, 4.21, 4.23
Nuclear pores, 4.21, 4.23
Nucleolus, 4.23
Nucleus, 3.1, 4.5, 4.23, 4.24, 5.1, 5.6
    skeletal muscle, 5.5
    smooth muscle, 2.21, 4.4

Oesophagus, 3.11, 3.20
Oestrogen, 5.18
Oligodendrocytes, 3.5, 5.6
Oocytes, 2.20, 4.1, 5.18
Open circulation model, 4.9
Optic vesicle, 5.14
Ora serrata, 1.19, 3.19
Ossification, 2.8, 4.8
Osteoblasts, 2.8, 4.8
Osteoclasts, 2.8, 5.2
Osteocytes, 2.8, 4.8
Osteoid, 4.8
Ovarian follicle, 2.20, 5.18
Ovary, 2.20, 5.18
Ovulation, 3.16
Ovum, 5.17, 5.18
Oxyphil cells, 4.15

Pacinian corpuscle, 2.7
Palatine tonsil, 2.11
Pancreas, 1.16, 3.12
Pancreatic ducts, 1.16, 3.12
Pancreatic polypeptide, 1.16, 3.12
Paneth cells, 2.12, 4.11, 4.12
Papilla of Vater, 3.12
Papillary (subpapillary) plexus, 5.8
Parasitic infection, 2.22
Parasympathetic ganglion cells, 1.14, 3.11
Parathyroid gland, 4.15
Parathyroid hormone, 2.8, 4.15
Parietal cells, 1.13, 4.11, 4.12, 5.13
Parotid glands, 1.12
Pedicels (foot processes), 3.24, 4.14
Penicillary arteries, 4.9
Pepsin, 4.11, 5.13
Pepsinogen, 5.13
Peptic (chief; zymogenic) cells, 1.13, 4.11, 5.13
Periarteriolar lymphoid sheath, 4.9
Pericardium, 1.8
Perichondrium, 1.9
Pericyte, 4.24